Waiting for Wings

A Woman's Metamorphosis Through Cancer

Heidi Marble

Foreword by James M. Long, MD

Ravenswood Court Publishing

ISBN: 978-1-885852-46-0
Library of Congress Control Number: 2006926110

The photographs in this book are by Heidi Neufeld Raine, Cordetta Spells, Mary Pat Reeves, Susan Campbell, Sharon Hanrahan, Henry Khoo, Vera Bogaerts, Jane Norton, Troy Marble and Heidi Marble, and are reproduced by permission.

Edited by Stephanie Parrish

Contact publisher through www.jspub.com.

DEDICATION

First and foremost, I thank my husband, Troy, for being my life partner. For your tenderness and devotion, and your wide-open heart.

My son, Blake. I started loving you even before you were born. You have an amazing, bright heart. Your life shines so much light and splendor. You are the best thing I have ever done.

My mom for raising me to believe in a higher power, to believe in myself and to see the goodness in all people. For showing me true courage and deep, unconditional love.

My grandmother, Wongee, for always living in the same house. For being the foundation I built my womanhood on. For your generous heart that always found a way to give to those in need.

My brother Justin Jon, who died too young, for teaching me about bugs and windshields. For being my guardian angel with an attitude. For showing me what a pure heart looks like. I miss you!

My dad, who died at fifty-nine, for showing me true grit. For your strength in the face of illness. For introducing me to horses, rodeos and cowgirl boots. For making me get back on after getting bucked off. For being fearless.

Be like the bird
That, pausing in her flight
Awhile on boughs too slight,
Feels them give way
Beneath her and yet sings,
Knowing that she hath wings.

Victor Hugo

Contents

FOREWORD

"I will survive!" This one phrase has characterized Heidi Marble's encounter with breast cancer. She was diagnosed at a very young age with inflammatory breast cancer. This is a virulent form of breast cancer that is fast growing and has a tendency to spread early and quickly. Heidi was determined to survive. She would survive for her child. She would survive for her husband. She would survive for herself. She did survive, against the odds, and at a great price. Then came the next hurdle: the need to heal and become whole.

At the end of the day, it is hope that sustains all of us, both patients and doctors. Doctors can help patients survive, and patients can help doctors survive. Hope is contagious. A patient says, "I don't want statistics. Just tell me, can I beat this thing? If so, tell me what we have to do, and let's get going!" I love this attitude! Hope is what it is all about.

I am often asked, "How do you deal every day with people who have cancer and not get down?" The answer, surprisingly, is this: the same people, those who have cancer, keep me cheered up. As a physician, I am often in awe of the men and women who have it set in their hearts that they will beat the cancer that has developed in their body. The path to survival demands a brave heart. Often the road is steep and the fatigue great. Of the hurdles met along the way, one of the greatest is the unspoken belief that cancer is unbeatable. If they listen to this siren song, it becomes easier to give up. "Tired? Just rest," they might hear. "Why fight? Nobody lives forever! Why put yourself and your family through all this?" Those who don't give in to these temptations but who maintain their pace without looking back are often the survivors. Truly it has been said, "Cancer isn't for wimps!"

Doctors themselves can sometimes harm patients by removing hope. A doctor says, "This disease is likely to kill you." What are you to think? You look at the wall of diplomas, the white coat and the gray hair. Are you going to disbelieve? But if you hear, "This cancer will be tough to beat, but it can be beat, and we will fight it together," you come away with a whole different feeling.

We are taught now that doctors shouldn't be fatherlike in their approach, telling patients what they should do. These days we are no longer called doctors and patients, but health-care providers and health-care consumers. Informed consent rules the day. Honesty is sometimes valued over compassion. The idea is to tell the patient the truth, what the options are and let them make a decision. Something has been lost in this translation. Truth can be harmful if it is not mixed with compassion and whatever honest hope that can be given.

Self-image is often instilled into us built by external forces. We live our lives playing the roles of who we think we are. Women are everywhere surrounded by displays of what others think it means to be a woman. They are almost overwhelmed by the variety and power of these images. Many women undertake similar journeys to a cure, which involve surgery, chemotherapy, radiation treatments and years of hormone therapy. Each step involves loss: the loss of the breast, the loss of hair, the loss of appetite, the loss of energy and the loss of self-image. Survival is one thing. It is one BIG thing. But after survival comes the next BIG thing: healing. The person who had cancer tries to become whole again.

The journey to healing is just as important as the one to the cure, and it is unique to each person. In *Waiting for Wings,* Heidi makes the journey through the valley of death and emerges whole. The things she had to give up on her journey cost her emotionally and physically, and she shares her feelings in the moving and emotional poetry she penned at the time. The message that emerges is that despite the loss of hair and the loss of breasts, a person can still be whole.

It is estimated that during the twelve months of 2006 in the United States alone, 212,920 new cases of breast cancer will be found. That equals 583 women each day. Your life will be touched by this disease. Whether it is yourself, your mother, your wife, your daughter or a coworker, you will know someone who has breast cancer. Learn from the insights shared in this book so that you can be a better friend to those who have to make this journey, be it yourself or someone else.

James M. Long, MD
Medical Director, North Bay Cancer Center

Acknowledgments

One page is too short to summarize the gratitude in my heart. I would like thank my amazing family and friends for being part of my life. To Heidi Raine, who initiated the idea of documenting my journey through photographs. For the huge role you played in my healing. To Cordetta Spells for your brilliant idea of a Buttons-n-Dollars fundraising campaign. For your world-class, Emmy Award-winning photography. For the countless hours you donated.

To Kathleen, Rachel and Susan for bringing me back to life. To Kimberly and Yasemin for traveling this journey with me. To Miss Frieda, my surrogate grandmother, for looking out for me. To Julie and Dan McQueen for the food, friendship and retreats at your home in Maine. To Marilyn, Julie's mom, who fought a brave battle with cancer. To the dynamic people at Hope Lodge in Massachusetts for helping those in need.

To Mary Pat for your fifteen-year friendship, love, humor and photographs. To Mr. Roger Dodger, friend since we were eleven and brother-in-law, for introducing me to your hairy-chested brother. For coming across the country to help us get through the diagnosis and surgery. For all the laughter and all your love. To Papa John and Mama John for being a source of strength. For keeping the house running and giving my mom a much-needed break.

To my Bay Area friends Alex & Kathie, Dana & Kelly, Scott & Jozie, Tom & Joan, Richard & Heidi, Vince & Michelle, Lee & Tonia, Phil & Kirsten for being my core. To Vivienne for being the daughter I never had. For helping me take care of my beautiful boy.

To my medical team from Boston all the way to Dr. James Long at North Bay Cancer Center. My life was in your hands and you have been an intricate part of fighting this disease. Also to North Bay Medical Center for believing in my cause of making a difference in the lives of people who deal with any kind of cancer and for giving me a platform to express my ideas.

To the Fairfield Center for the Creative Arts for supporting my artistic endeavors. A big hug for Andrea Garcia, features writer extraordinaire, for so thoughtfully expressing my story in the *Daily Republic*. Mr. Ezio Lucido and Company at Motion Eclipse Pictures for creating a documentary that blew my mind and for the meaningful, rich conversations we've shared.

To Greg and James at Graphic Auto Body in Fairfield for being willing to step out of the box to paint my mannequins.

Deep gratitude to Jim Stevenson, my publisher, for making my dream a reality.

For expanding your genre just for me. To editing angel Stephanie Parrish, not only for your precise skills, but also for your compassion. To my marketing friend Jerry Jinette for helping me devise a plan to create a business based on my belief of helping others first.

Introduction

Wings of any kind have always fascinated me, whether on the back of a butterfly or a graceful lark. Wings elevate the body to new heights, allowing us to see from a different perspective. The world becomes larger and more full of possibilities as we elevate ourselves. Where we land is our choice; where we fly becomes our destiny.

Not all creatures that now soar with their wings were born with them. The butterfly is one. The process it must undergo to develop them is difficult, even painful. Before a caterpillar becomes a butterfly, it becomes very restless. It may leave the plants that have always been its home to find a safe place to undergo its transformation. When the caterpillar finds the right spot, it weaves a silk foundation on a twig or leaf. There it attaches itself and hangs upside down, and waits. During this stage the caterpillar is at rest. Finally, when the time is right, it begins moving vigorously, forcing the casing to open. It struggles for hours to shed the old layer of skin. When the skin is gone, the caterpillar looks like a large green water drop. Then its shape and color begin to change. The outer layer hardens into an stunning emerald case, decorated with gold specks. Inside this chrysalis, miraculous things are happening. Soon the outer shell becomes transparent enough for the butterfly within to be seen. When the butterfly emerges, its wings are wrinkled and wet, and it clings desperately to the cocoon. If the emergence is interrupted or hurried, the fluid from the abdomen of the butterfly will never be pushed into its wings. It will spend the rest of its life with a swollen abdomen and shriveled wings, unable to fly. This book, *Waiting for Wings*, explains my own metamorphosis. This is the journey of my transformation from the edge of death to the sky above.

April 12 was the day, 2000 was the year. The morning was crisp and bright in our sleepy New England town of Grafton, forty miles west of Boston. Smooth, green hills studded with sheep and nostalgic farms were the backdrop. I opened the bedroom window just a crack and the warm breeze lifted the hem of my lace curtain. The sharp edge of winter was finally pulling away. I entered my bathroom and started to get ready for another doctor's appointment. My two-year-old son was at my feet. His chattering and giggles filled the air with joyful sounds. I did my hair and put my makeup on with fractured attention. Blake was full of energy and on a mission to find whatever might have been dropped on the floor. I picked him up in my arms and he nestled his head on my chest. I grabbed my purse, car keys, a baggy of Goldfish crackers, and out the door we went. I dropped Blake off at my friend Kathleen's house. He wobbled over to the sandbox and started to push a small bulldozer in the sand, making sputtering sounds with his lips.

I made it to Belmont Street. The parking lot was full, so I took the opportunity to sing my favorite Eagles song. Finally, I found the perfect spot under a barren maple tree. For some reason, I paused and took notice of the branches that were pregnant with leaves. One final lipstick check in the rearview mirror and I was ready.

Quickly, I entered the old brick building; the sterile smell was a stark contrast from the fresh air. I struggled with the heavy, brown door and its uncooperative handle. The front desk greeted me with a clipboard full of papers. Insurance cards were copied and I plopped down in a stiff chair. I began riffling through out-of-date magazines; the most pressing thing on my mind was what I would cook for dinner.

Six months prior, while bending over to get a pair of shoes in my closet, I noticed some isolated pain in the upper-left quadrant of my breast. The succession of appointments offered various benign explanations: fibrocystic breast changes, too much caffeine, residual changes from breast-feeding. This all seemed logical, until I started to lose weight and was blanketed by fatigue. At thirty-four years old, with a clean mammography reading only fourteen months prior, no one seemed impressed with my symptoms. Somehow, deep inside, I sensed something was terribly wrong with my body. I started to question my own instincts with each uneventful inquiry. Then my breast started to swell and red streaks appeared.

It was six o'clock in the evening when I decided to leave a voice mail for the surgeon I had consulted with a few years back. The phone rang and rang, until I heard an irritated male voice on the line. He was grumbling about his secretary forgetting to turn on the answering machine. I realized Dr. Quinlan was on the phone with me. It was nothing less than divine intervention that he picked up the call. He asked me to come in the following day, suspecting I had a serious infection.

Back to the waiting room. The nurse finally called my name and led me to a small examination room. I changed into a starched, worn-out gown and loosely tied the frayed straps behind my shoulders. I hopped up on the examination table, my sweaty hands sticking to the paper. I felt like a deli sandwich waiting to be wrapped. Posters of cross-sectioned breasts made me cringe. Two knocks at the door and Dr. Quinlan entered, while thumbing through my thin medical chart. Small talk ensued until he pulled down the corner of my gown to reveal my breast. His eyes grew large and then intense with focus. He ordered his nurse to retrieve a biopsy kit. With distinct terminology, he stated the two possible diagnoses: 1) an infection or 2) a rare, deadly form of breast cancer. He sunk the needle deep into the hardest part of my breast. Then the nurse cleaned and dressed the wounds before I was rushed to mammography across the street. All the while I was telling myself, it's just an infection. I can't have cancer. I'm too young. I have a child to raise!

The mammography machine was unforgiving as it pressed my bleeding breast into a pancake. The technician was quiet and would not indulge in my attempts at small talk. Next came the ultrasound machine. I looked at the screen with all of its gray, wavy lines and didn't notice anything scary. I figured that with some high-potency antibiotics, the problem would be solved! Back to another examination room, more deli paper, more posters and more old magazines. Two knocks again; this time Dr. Quinlan entered slowly with a young female doctor. Her coat was pressed smooth, and my eyes were drawn to the word embroidered above her pocket: "Oncologist." Before they had a chance to say a word, I whispered, "I have cancer, don't I?" As they confirmed, they moved closer and held me, while I broke into pieces. They helped me stand and led me down a long corridor to view the X-rays. I heard the glass doors slide open behind me, and my husband, Troy, was standing there. I ran to him, held him close and said, "I have cancer"; his only response was NO!

In the dimly lit room, the mammogram films were neatly lined up in two rows. Dr. Quinlan's words felt like bullets as he proceeded to point out the deadly calcifications, too numerous to count. In what seemed like a foreign language, he fired off a battle plan.

1. More tests to see if the cancer had spread to the brain, liver, lungs or bones
2. Echocardiogram to make sure my heart was strong enough to endure high-dose chemotherapy
3. Surgery to insert a portacath into my chest for the administration of high-dose chemotherapy
4. If the treatment reduced the size of the breast to an operable state, a radical mastectomy
5. Based on pathology results, the possibility of a bone marrow transplant
6. High-dose radiation treatments followed by hormonal therapy
7. Lupron injections to shut down my ovaries and reduce my estrogen level

My only question was, how much time do you think I have? He hesitated and said that due to the fact that I had inflammatory breast cancer, I was looking at approximately eighteen months. He explained that this particular cancer creates layers or nests, causing swelling and pain, and often involves the skin. It spreads almost like a virus. It is very aggressive. In those suspended moments, I felt like a part of me died. My future ran like water on thirsty ground, just disappearing. My chemotherapy was scheduled to begin four days later.

Within thirteen days, my hair was gone. I was stripped of my beauty and all signs of life. The first time I saw my bald image, I thought I looked like a worm. That seemed too harsh, so I decided that comparing myself to a caterpillar was better. It was then that I knew I would need to go through a metamorphosis, whether into survival or death; in either case change was coming. My cocoon would be created with hope, love, prayers and plenty of chocolate.

An amazing friend, who is also named Heidi, offered to document my journey through photographs. I wanted to leave a lasting testimony of my fight to stay alive so that one day my son would understand that I did not leave him willingly. Our photo sessions, although serious in nature, ended up being a source of fun. I sat half naked in trees, giant nests and on hard bricks with plants around my head just to get the perfect shot. The most powerful picture she took is the one with the words "I Will Survive" written on my back with eyeliner. This was my declaration for life. All the while, I would turn to my black journal and pour my feelings into words and poetry, never realizing a book was being born.

Six years later, I come to you cancer free. *Waiting for Wings* takes you through my transformation from despair to hope. Intertwined throughout the book are photographs, journal entries and various insights. The photography is a blend of the artistry of several amazing friends who have so lovingly documented my metamorphosis. You will see references to nests, birds and butterflies, which were my delicate reminders of hope. My cocoon had my husband's unconditional love, my son's amazing laughter, my family's devotion, my friends' acceptance, thousands of prayers, cards and letters, the compassion of the medical world and the strength of my fellow travelers. I moved away from everything I knew, attached myself to a safe place and became quiet. My chrysalis hardened to protect the vulnerable being inside. When the time was right, I became restless and came out, never rushing the process. I emerged with my first burst of color. All the love, pain and suffering were pushed into my shriveled wings. I could feel them unfolding, lifting the weight I had carried for so long. My wish for you is that your struggles will elevate you into your potential. There is nothing more powerful than realizing you've had your wings all along.

WAITING FOR WINGS

If I could wrap myself in silken string
Create warmth and shelter out of pain
I'd hide away in this cocoon
Waiting for wings

Instead
I crawl naked and colorless
Uncertainty threatens to pluck me away

I envision the rapture of emerging
Light drying the wetness of my rebirth

I'll unfold my wings
Step to the edge
Float with the wind

I won't need to look up
For I will have already touched the sky

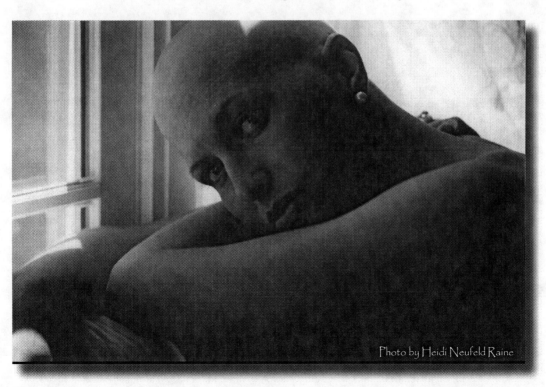

Photo by Heidi Neufeld Raine

Part One
Diagnosis, Hair
Loss
and
Chemotherapy

Photo by Heidi Neufeld Raine

Within four days of my diagnosis, I entered the world of chemotherapy. The doctors gave me high doses of Cytoxin with an IV push of Adriamicin. The Adriamicin caused my urine to turn red—an unpleasant surprise. When the chemotherapy was first administered, I felt a cold burning sensation. I could actually taste it, and the odor seemed to fill my nostrils. I just kept trying to imagine the medication as a gold light that was healing my body. It was difficult to embrace something so punishing.

The medication dripped for over three hours, every moment feeling like an eternity. All around me, people sat in various-colored recliners, forced to look at each other. Most were extremely quiet and expressionless, but one woman cried out, "I can't take it anymore!" The nurses rushed to console her and to encourage her to keep going. During that suspension in hell, I stared at a picture of my two-year-old son, Blake, in his yellow overalls, with his toothless grin. I finally understood what people mean when they say they'll do anything for their children. I was willing to undergo any pain or side effects, if more time with him was possible.

It didn't get bad until later in the evening. That is when the cramping started and the scent of chemotherapy overtook me. I went upstairs alone and took a shower to try to get rid of the smell, but nothing could mask the saturation. Quiet tears came as I laid down. I touched my hair over and over again, noticing its softness, length and sweet smell, trying to imagine what it would be like to be bald. It didn't take long for the tranquilizers to do their job, and I fell asleep.

About thirteen days later, when my hair started to fall out, my hairstylist, Stacy, suggested that I cut my hair shorter every few days. This would allow me to adjust to the baldness gradually. When my hair was ear length, I asked Stacy if she would be willing to shave my hair at my house. At this point, I could pull out huge bundles with very little effort. She asked me to bend my head over, and I heard the clippers come on. She started at the base of my skull and made one huge stripe from the back of my head to the front. My hair was falling all around me, sliding down the slippery, black cape onto the floor. When Stacy was finished, I felt my head and its intermittent stubble. I had the sensation of feeling exposed and naked. I looked at my bald head in the small mirror and surprisingly felt some relief that it was finally over. My husband broke the silence by saying, "Ha, ha, you thought I would go bald first."

I carefully considered ahead of time how I would introduce Blake to his mother's baldness. I bought various silly wigs and hats at a costume shop and hid them away. When the time came, I put on a turban and a hat. Blake's first instinct was to remove the hat and then the turban. I just went with the flow. "Mommy looks funny, huh?" I told him I was taking magic medicine and that I could have any kind of hair I wanted. His blue eyes were wide and his mouth open. I put on the clown wig and then Rapunzel and of course some dreadlocks. Before I knew it, he had wigs on too and we were laughing.

Prior to going bald, I purchased a wig that was supposed to look like my own hair. Boy was I in for a surprise! Immediately, the wig and I had serious issues. It was either too tight or too loose. I couldn't stand the white foam head that came with it. The wig also had an odor that is hard to describe. My attempts to style it only led to frustration. Once, I overcurled the wig and ended up throwing it on the shower floor. I squirted a huge glob of shampoo and took out my anger on this defenseless prosthesis. When I was done flinging it around and crying, I hung it up on the shower caddy to dry.

Wig wearing became a "special occasion" event. The rest of the time, I opted for soft scarves, turbans and cute hats. When I did wear the wig, I had about an hour time limit. At that point, it was usually passed around by friends who took great pleasure in trying it on.

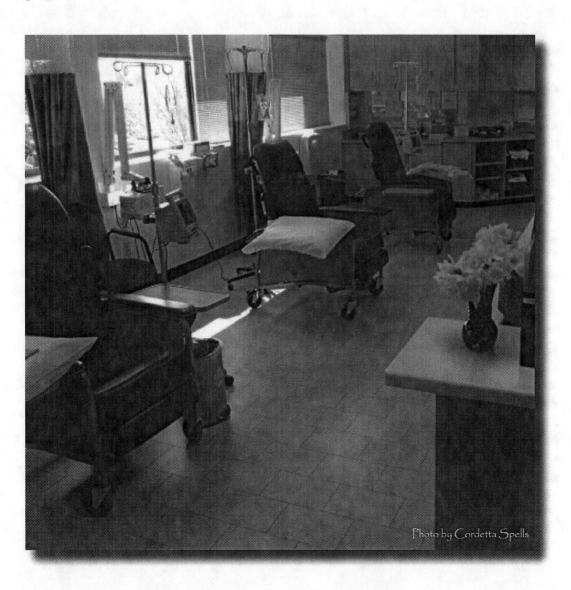

Photo by Cordetta Spells

UMass Memorial/Memorial Campus
Diagnostic Imaging
Memorial Campus
119 Belmont Street
Worcester MA 01605

MRN: 000671363

Attending Physician:
Address: 291 LINCOLN STREET

WORCESTER, MA   01605

Patient: MARBLE, HEIDI
DOB: 30-Sep-1965
Visit Number:

Acc#: 3735900   Exam: MAMMO DX BILAT

Exam Date: 12-Apr-2000 11:15 AM

Requester: Memorial, Doctor

Status: D
Location:

Patient type: OUT-PATIENT

History/Clinical Data:
STRONG HX OF BREAST CANCER MOTHER, GRANDMOTHER, GREAT GRANDMOTHER. P
AIN AND TENDERNESS ON THE LEFT.

Phys: QUINLAN,ROBERT   Req: QUINLAN,ROBERT

Bilateral mammography compared to a study of 9/11/98. Again, the
breasts are extremely dense and lesion could be missed with this
type of breast parenchyma. No change in the appearance of the
right breast is noted.

On the left, there has been a marked change with the presence on
the current examination of innumerable microcalcifications.
Findings are consistent with the clinical impression of an
inflammatory carcinoma. By history, a needle biopsy of the area
has already been performed. Films reviewed with Dr. Quinlan.

BI-RADS CATEGORY 5:
Highly suggestive of malignancy.

(2a)

d - 4/12/00
m - 4/14/00

Dictated By: Millard, Jack R., M.D.

Transcribed By: Conversion, Data   Date: 1-Jul-2000   7:30 AM
Finalized By: MILLARD, JACK R., M.D.   Date: 1-Jul-2000   7:30 AM

DOOR TO HELL

Newborn leaves cast their shadows
April 12 on Belmont Street
An examination room waits
I take the stairs one flight up
Air stale and medical

I am told to undress
In glass jars, instruments marinate
The table is old Styrofoam
Paper sticks to my hands
Two polite knocks at the door
He enters with his knowledge well groomed
Examines my angry breast
Black bifocals balance on a dignified nose
Worry crumples his brow
He asks for the hollow needle
Sinks it deep
I rattle and coil
His nurse begins to cry

At the machine, I pose
Breast smashed between plates
I wipe blood and wait
He enters again
Helps me stagger down the hall
And opens the door to hell

Low-lit mammogram films line the wall
Purgatory's decoration
Malignant calcifications are sprinkled like sand
Too many to count

Hands skilled at cutting hold mine
Sharp blue eyes soften
Inferno's symphony plays
I begin my dance with the devil

Photos by Heidi Marble

CANCER'S BALLET

Position one
Catheter in my chest
Snagged with a crooked needle
Catch of the day

Position two
Deliberate drugs infuse
Through the clear snake on my lap

Position Three
Hours stagnate
Pharmaceuticals make their way to every pore
I am steeped in it

Position Four
The needle is pulled from the plastic jaw
I am released

Position Five
I find a hollow toilet
Pirouette on a frigid tile stage
Hold the metal bar
Urinate crimson and plié into hell

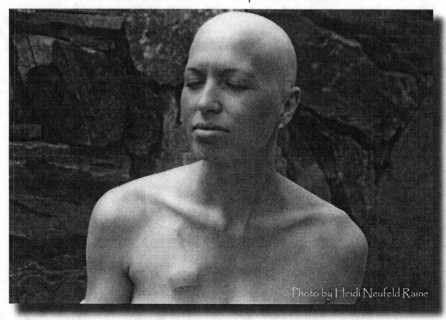

Photo by Heidi Neufeld Raine

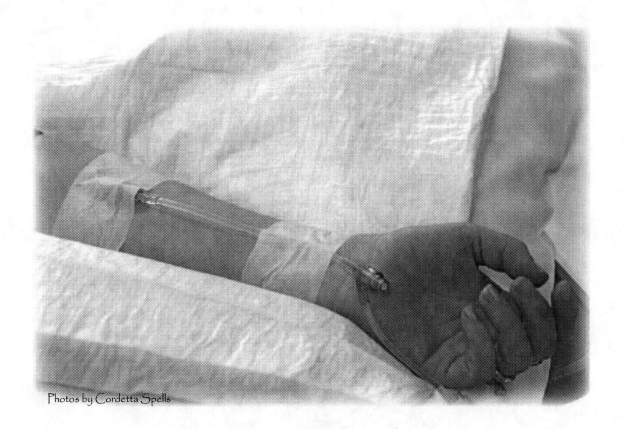

Photos by Cordetta Spells

SHAVED

Golden tresses clog the drain
Exhausted follicles itch
My pillowcase smothered with strands

I bow at the altar of cancer
Make my first sacrifice
The shaver leaves a naked trail
The room breathes on my scalp

What used to flow and spill
Lies quiet beside me on the floor
I scrape a razor against the stubble
Rub in warm lotion with my hands
Touch the rawness with apprehension
Collect my hair as a souvenir

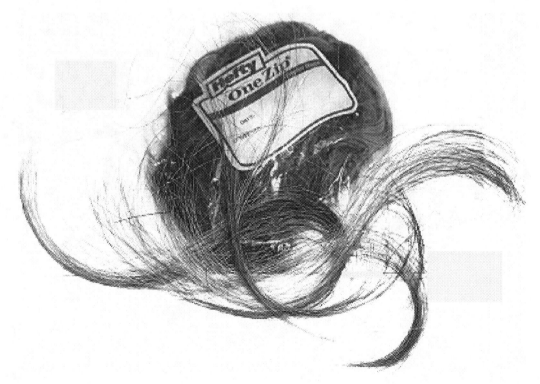

Photo by Heidi Neufeld Raine

STRAWBERRY MOON

Water closes around me
The tub holds my weary body
A candle flame moves in time with my breath
The arched faucet drools
My single ounce of strength shuts it off
I explore my baldness
Accepting, denying
Summer moon beckons behind the shade
June has blessed the ground with berries
Deep and red
Water beads on my skin
I enter the night
Let the towel fall
Bathe in illumination
Balmy air engulfs me

Photo by Heidi Neufeld Raine

ESCAPE

In my mind
I see a checkered blanket
My hair gold and streaming
I am in repose

The sky blue and billowing with clouds
Birds sing
The breeze moves my white gauze dress
Summer brown skin
Sweet perfume

A butterfly opens and shuts its papery wings
A ripe peach drips sweet juice into my mouth
Sprawling trees dance and sing
Flowers turn their faces to the sun
Water runs over smooth rocks
I dangle my feet in the stream
Pull blades of grass through my fingers and dream

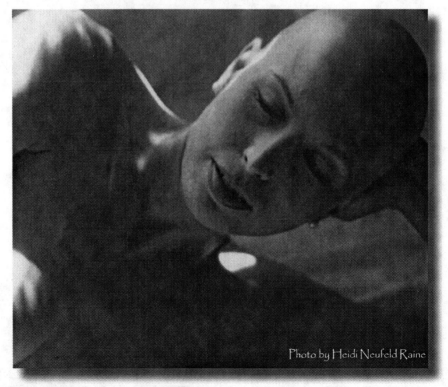

Photo by Heidi Neufeld Raine

CIRCUS

Here for your fascination
Under the big top
Painted-on smile, neon wig
I juggle relentlessly
Mime my words
In a cage with the lion, my whip cracks
He bears his long, white teeth
I walk a tightrope, with no net below
Trapped animals wait their turn
Elephants sit up like poodles getting a treat
Children stare tasting their cotton-candy fingers
Drum roll please
I'm ready to go home

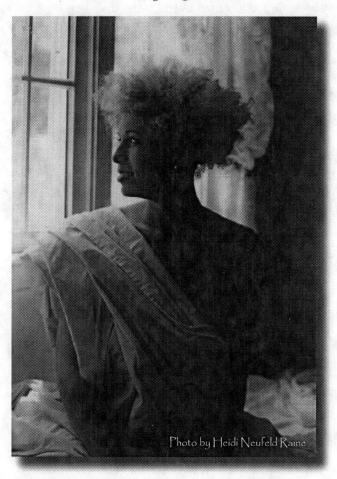

Photo by Heidi Neufeld Raine

VOID

My brush sits idle
Still wrapped with blonde hair

No use for lavender shampoo
I cancel the hairdresser
Barrettes are banished to the bottom drawer

I remove the pins from her Styrofoam head
Release the wig, fumble with the straps
My scalp resents the tightness

Pack the last of my pretty ribbons
Her expression remains void
While I clean hair off my rollers

I hate her purpose
As if one bald head isn't enough
Inanimate voyeur
Witness to my devastation

I peel the wig off my head
Deep, red indentations remaining
Now it's her turn to wear the wig

I carry her to my closet
Shove her face first against the wall
She deserves the darkness

Photo by Heidi Neufeld Raine

DESPAIR'S BANQUET

Despair sets her table with fine linen
Sharp utensils at her plate
Wax drips from black candles
A dusty chandelier dimly lighting her table
The dinner bell rings

She picks me up with her spindly fingers
Runs her tongue over dry lips
The aroma of my weakness whetting her appetite

She loves pain raw
It does not matter that I am frozen and thin
She eats anyway
She takes her portions large
Taking seconds on my dreams

My body her banquet
My blood her brandy
My hope her leftovers

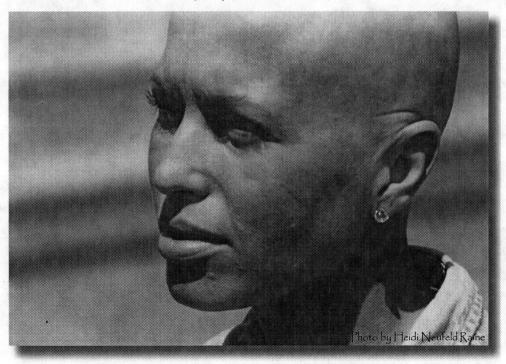

Photo by Heidi Neufeld Raine

MOSAIC SOUL

Shoved off a high shelf
I fall and shatter
In millions of little pieces
My edges are sharp and uneven
Nothing seems to fit
There are just stark white spaces hardening too fast

I need an artist
With thick plaster and design
Who will wipe the residue away
Showing me where I begin
Where I end

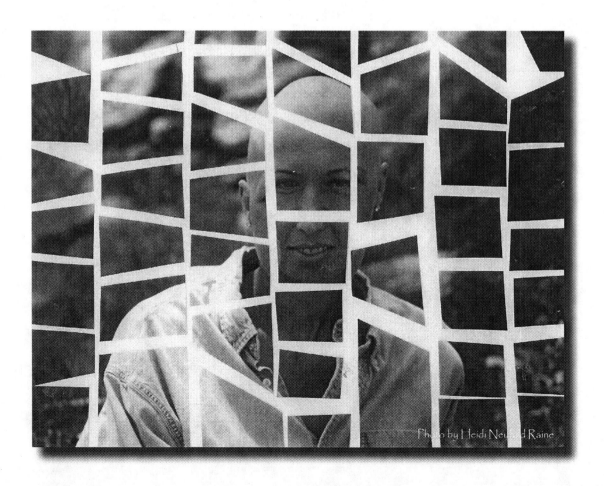

Photo by Heidi Neu and Raine

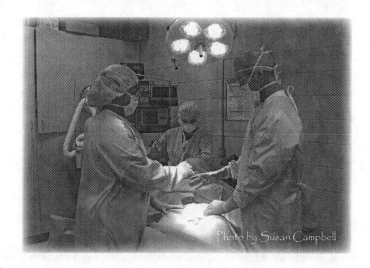

Photo by Susan Campbell

Part Two
Surgery

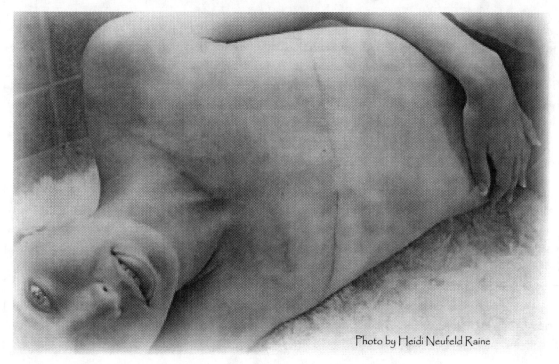

Photo by Heidi Neufeld Raine

On my diagnosis day, it was suggested to me that I consider having a portacath inserted. Initially, I thought it had something to do with urination. As it turned out, that might have been more appealing. This device is placed under the skin in the chest, and a tube is inserted into a main artery, allowing high doses of chemotherapy to be administered. In addition, it was supposed to be less painful than the numerous needle sticks that I would have had otherwise. I reluctantly consented and went in for this outpatient surgery.

When I woke up, it was a lot more uncomfortable than I had expected. After arriving home, I carefully inspected my new friend. It was ugly; it looked like there was a contact lens case with a leash under my skin. You could clearly see the contraption along with its tube. It was repulsive to look at this new addition to my chest. Ultimately, I learned to adjust and was relieved to be able to receive the medication I needed without additional suffering.

By the time my second chemotherapy was over, my breast was shrinking. I was having what the medical field calls a dramatic response to chemotherapy. During my follow-up visit, my surgeon felt that in two more rounds I should be ready to have my breast removed. I couldn't wait to get rid of my breast. I know that sounds funny, but I wanted it gone. It was threatening my life and my well-being. I was constantly examining whether or not it was continuing to shrink. My poor female friends got to see my breast on a regular basis to look for improvement as well.

I decided on a female breast surgeon named Dr. Sue Troyan at Beth Israel Deaconess Hospital in Boston. She was willing to embrace my need to remove my healthy breast too. It was a rock-solid decision for me not to have to end up with cancer in the other breast and enduring all of this again. Because of the aggressive nature of my cancer, she agreed. She also encouraged me to wait on reconstruction until my body regained its strength. Building breasts out of other parts of my body didn't and doesn't seem very appealing. At that time and now, minimally painful surveillance for cancer's recurrence and survival top my list. To date, I am still not ready to undergo reconstructive surgery because of the possible complications.

I spent the next few weeks saying good-bye to this part of my femininity. I reflected back on all the silly exercises I did as a teenager to encourage my breasts to grow. I recalled the first time my mom took me to buy a bra. I laughed remembering how I said "size zero" when the saleslady asked my cup size. I remembered the hours I spent nursing Blake and the amazing feeling that came with nourishing my baby. I thought about all the bathing suits and clothes I would no longer be able to fill out. I thought about how it will feel for Troy to see this part of my body gone. I worried because I knew he wasn't a leg man! I contemplated how I would handle this loss. I considered the three-inch spread of numbness that would soon take over my chest. I spent time looking in the mirror, smashing my breasts with my hands, trying to imagine their absence. The afternoon before my surgery, I went through all of my bras and packed them up for donation. I cried when I folded each one and placed it in a cardboard box. The last night I had my breasts, I took a bath alone and said my final farewell. I never touched them again.

The surgery was early in the morning on July 18. I was weak and ravaged by chemotherapy. Pre-op went smoothly. Dr. Troyan comforted me and went on her way to scrub. Nurses brought me pleasure in their needles, and the next thing I remember were voices telling me to breathe. There was talk of not enough oxygen and of bleeding, but I couldn't open my eyes yet. I felt someone messing with my left side. A few moments later, I woke because of the persistent prodding. Four hours in recovery and I was finally ready for a room. On the way, I started vomiting from the anesthesia; luckily, that didn't last long. My chest was tightly wrapped, and I had four grenade-shaped drains, two on each side, to help draw fluid from the surgical sites. Then they had these ridiculous blow-up contraptions on my legs to prevent blood clots. Between the beeping, blowing and monitoring, sleep was hard to come by.

At 9:00 the next morning, Dr. Troyan came in to check the wounds. She ran the curtain around the track and started to carefully unwrap the dressings. With deep compassion she introduced me to my flat chest. Shortly thereafter, a sweet lady entered with two huge cotton bra stuffers. Apparently, they only had size D's left; they looked like footballs. I wasn't willing to walk out of the hospital bald and skinny with two enormous mounds of obviously fake breasts. She politely packed them in a "booby bag" for me so I could wear them later.

Within twenty-seven hours after surgery, I was discharged from the hospital. At home, I felt broken and unable to rally. Troy put a lock on the upper part of our door so I could deal with my drains in privacy. For days, I could hear life down below in the kitchen and family room. The unfairness of the situation was starting to get to me. Ten days later, I had the drains removed--I could have done without that procedure. On the count of three, Dr. Troyan yanked out what seemed like three feet of tubing from each side. Afterward, it was wonderful to be free from the burden of carrying them around.

Before I even finished healing from surgery, more high-dose chemotherapy started. This time I would take it really hard. The drug Taxol numbed my feet, my fingertips and part of my lip. It made my bones ache to the point that I needed narcotics to cope. My joints became stiff, my desire for food left, and I had to endure additional injections to keep my blood count from plummeting too low. I was barely functional at this point, my balance was terrible, and I was weak from anemia. My skin was covered with bruises and my mouth was riddled with sores. I understood that I was teetering on the edge of death. There was a time we had gone to Cape Cod directly after my treatment that I even considered ending my life. I was heavily drugged and not thinking clearly. I stepped into the ocean, and it felt like an invitation to let go. I was up to my neck in water when I heard my son laugh from a hundred yards away. His laugh snapped me back into reality. I turned around and made my way back to the shore. I collapsed on the sand, overwhelmed with grief.

In the midst of all of this pain, my curious mind was ticking away. I wanted to know what became of my breasts. If a funeral for them would be in order? Maybe little headstones? It seemed odd that a part of my body was gone without a proper send-off. After I discovered their fate, (they were cross-sectioned and frozen for research), I stopped making inquiries of this nature.

CUT AWAY

Tomorrow they'll be gone
Cut away
Steely tools wait on blue paper
Shiny
Until my body weeps blood
In the bureaucracy of paperwork
I sign repeatedly
Until the divorce of my flesh is finalized
Custody awarded to curious doctors
Who divide my breasts amongst themselves
My husband grieves the pending separation
Wets my chest with tears
I pull him close to my heart
Feel him break
The time has come
Hospital jewelry on my wrist
Medication placates
Next in line
I count backward into unconsciousness

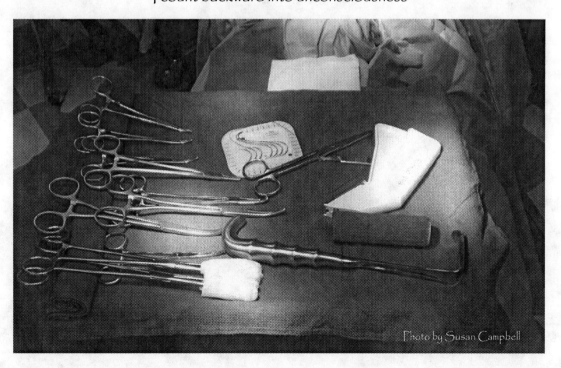

Photo by Susan Campbell

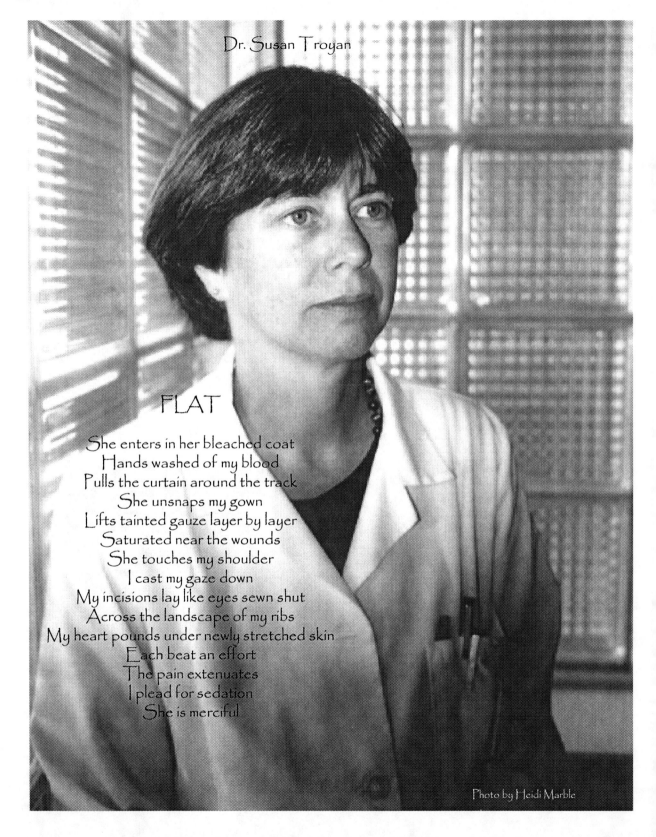

Dr. Susan Troyan

FLAT

She enters in her bleached coat
Hands washed of my blood
Pulls the curtain around the track
She unsnaps my gown
Lifts tainted gauze layer by layer
Saturated near the wounds
She touches my shoulder
I cast my gaze down
My incisions lay like eyes sewn shut
Across the landscape of my ribs
My heart pounds under newly stretched skin
Each beat an effort
The pain extenuates
I plead for sedation
She is merciful

Photo by Heidi Marble

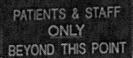

PATIENTS & STAFF
ONLY
BEYOND THIS POINT

THE DEPTH OF SUMMER

Plugged in like an appliance
Each pulse recorded
Skullcap moist with perspiration
Gurney wheeled recklessly
My feet are so cold
Pale pink bedpan in my hands
Drains nuzzle my sides like nursing puppies
Edgy nurses whisper
Tuck me into stiff white sheets
No bedtime story here
A large fluorescent light buzzes
The chain is out of reach
Morphine dispenses every eleven minutes
I hear the machine push the dose
I watch the drip reach my hand
I feel it intermingle with my blood
My eyes stagger to stay open
I fold my arms over my wounded chest
Family stands at the foot of my bed
Pain reflects back in their eyes
Outside the window
Summer lives without me

Photo by Heidi Neufeld Raine

WHY ME?

Why did you choose me?
Was my soul on its last breath?
Did the abandoned pain turn into insidious hungry cells?
Did I feel too much, then not enough?
I can't recall the sound of my laughter
Did it fill the air like my son's?
All I know now are the traces of scalpels
Long and numb
Where my heart used to be

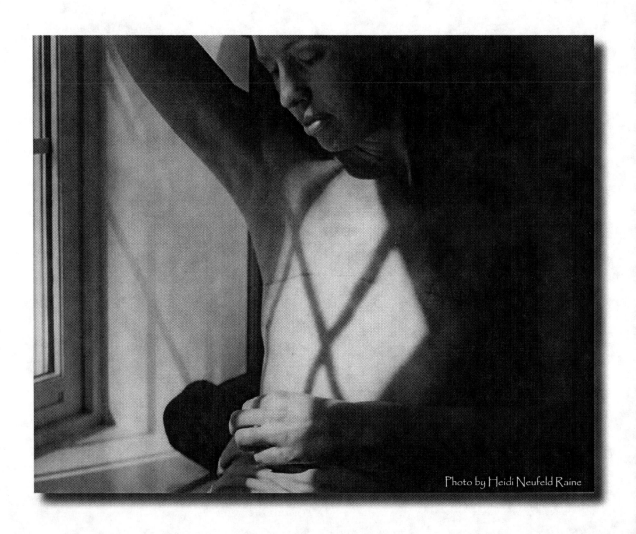

Photo by Heidi Neufeld Raine

DONATION

Hangers swing
I drop my life, dress by dress
Into the mouth of a cardboard box
IF
I could dance one more time in black lace
IF
I could stretch lycra over an expectant belly
IF
I could twirl in red satin
Dine in royal blue
Walk the beach in ivory silk
IF
I could go back
IF
I could remember the softness of my flesh
Trace perfume down my cleavage

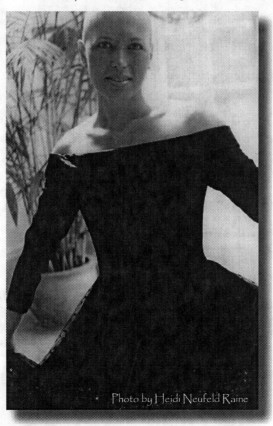

Photo by Heidi Neufeld Raine

TANGLED

Invited by the ocean's voice
I lift myself from ashen sand
Part my mouth, indulge in the breeze's salty kiss
Chemotherapy fresh in my veins
Narcotics stupefy

The water is frigid and wild
I step in
Tired of the tangled net
The pounding surf
I go deeper into nature's mouth

The cold waves numb me
I imagine my last exhalation
Sinking into stillness
I shut my tired eyes
I start to let go
Then I hear my son laugh in the distance
I am reeled back to the shore
Anchored

Photo by Troy Marble

DISGUISE

Alabaster canvas, water-stained mirror
I pull open my makeup drawer
Paint my lips cinema pink
Twist the color back in the tube
Black mascara is dry
Wand covered with fallen lashes
I line my naked eyelids smoky brown
Dust my cheekbones fresh peach
Cover bruises with concealer
Thick and dark
Cover my legs with pants
Baggy and wide
Select a scarf
Tie it around my head
Push my earrings into each hole
My wedding ring is too loose
I hide it away
Run a file over brittle nails
Streaks of dried blood underneath
I paint them Valentine red
Shut off the bathroom lights
Count to ten and try to find the beauty
Tired of seeking
I hide

Photo by Heidi Neufeld Raine

EMACIATED

Buried alive
In this flesh-and-bone coffin
The depth so profound
Do I want to emerge?
Dampness seeps through my skin
I am chilled to the core
Pain eclipses any light
Through a sheer, black veil
I see a velvet-lined box
A blue, satin pillow
A single rose in my lifeless hands
I long for eternal rest
I want to seep away
Like water in search of its end

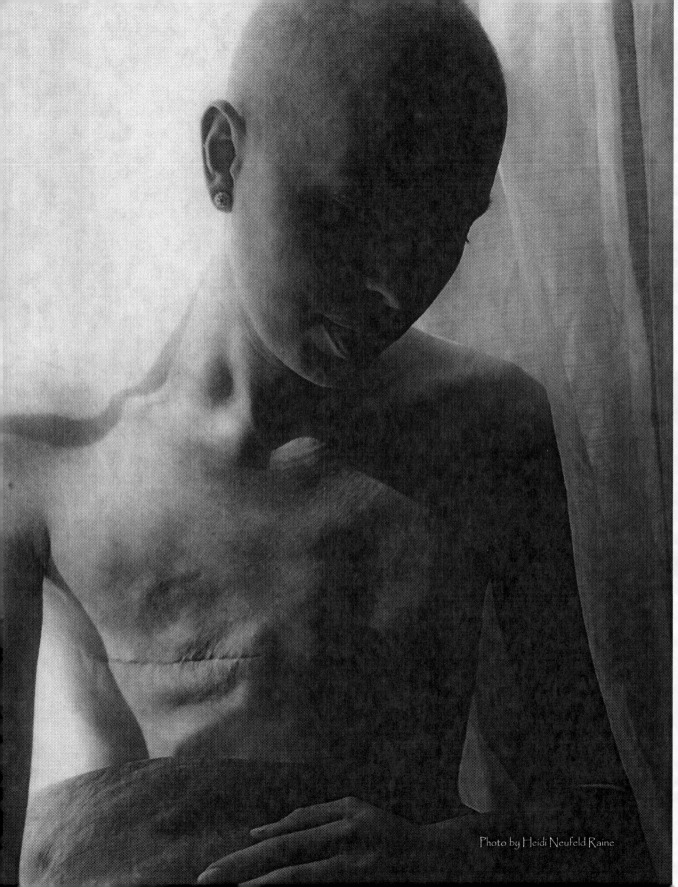

Photo by Heidi Neufeld Raine

HUNTED

A canopy of fear stifles the sun
I am paralyzed
Startled
Each blink sustained
The future no longer expansive
My life miscarried

The beast follows my scent
Fondles the air with wide nostrils
Branches crack
The unknown lurks

Will I be spared?
Will I be silenced?
Will I fight?
Will I succumb?

VAMPIRES' SURVEILLANCE

The rubber tourniquet tightly pulled
The steel needle rests in the top of my hand
I wait in vampires' kitchen while
Syringes drink to capacity
Vials contain the verdict
I am tempted to break them
Write "Helter Skelter" on sterile walls
Run until I catch the dreams I've lost
Instead
I sit
Each ring of the phone crawls up my spine
I imagine vampires spinning the blood
Rocking it back and forth
Microscopes zoom
While I wait
And wait
And wait

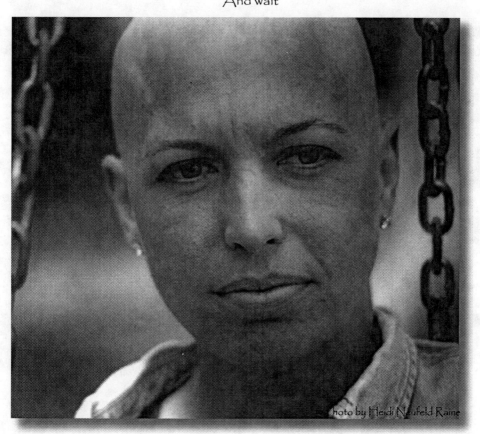

photo by Heidi Neufeld Raine

BOOBS FOR SALE

Saleslady with a tidy briefcase
Full of ABC's
Asks me which size I prefer

She explains the warranty
Unfolds the white pocket bra
Slips the prosthesis in

She takes my American Express
I sign in the glare of her sealed-deal smile
Cross breasts off my shopping list

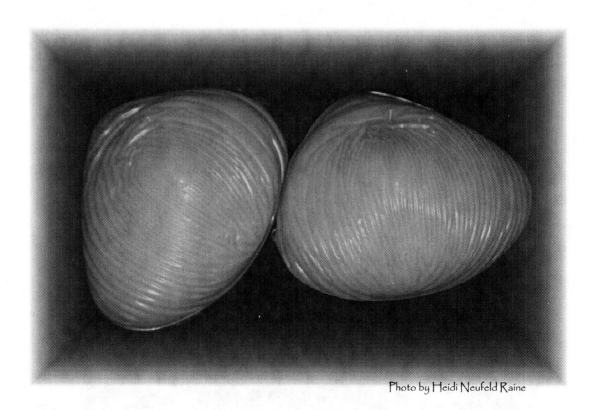

Photo by Heidi Neufeld Raine

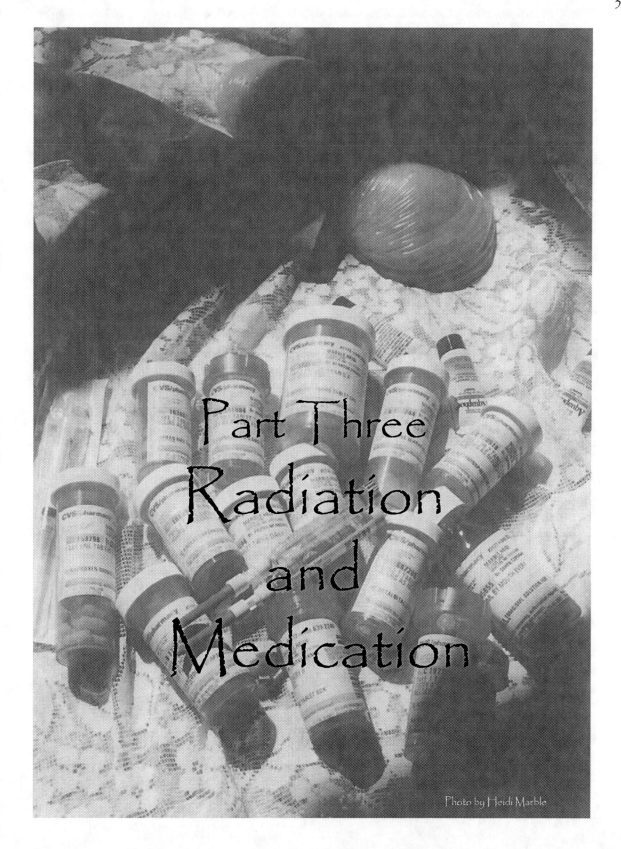

Part Three
Radiation
and
Medication

Photo by Heidi Marble

Radiation was a surreal experience that happened five days a week for almost two months. After my final chemotherapy treatment, I went into the dungeons of the hospital for my first radiation appointment. I sat with a nurse for forty-five minutes as she explained the possible side-effects and remedies. Then I went for a spiral CT scan so they could do three-dimensional mapping. This would enable them to accurately target the radiation and preserve as much healthy tissue as possible. It wasn't long until a nice gentleman came out and gave me my tattoos. I requested something more creative than black spots; he just laughed. The tattoos would serve as a dot-to-dot alignment grid.

A few days later, I returned to the basement level of the hospital. The nurse assigned a locker for my clothes and gave me another worn-out gown to wear. I then sat in the waiting room with a bunch of men who had lost their sense of modesty. Apparently, they had become immune to the world above us. Their biggest concern was getting through the riggers of radiation; soon I followed suit.

Finally, it was my turn, and I entered a huge room with enormous equipment. The shelves were lined with brain-radiation masks that looked like string-covered faces. On the opposite side, the molds to hold each patient's position were hanging with our names written on the outside. My mold was placed on the hard table. I disrobed and was manually adjusted until the laser beams aligned. I asked them to play "Calling All Angels" on the CD player. I knew the song would last as long as the treatment. If I could just get lost in the song then maybe I could disengage from the reality of being burned.

The technicians stepped behind a thick wall and talked to me on some type of speaker that initially scared the daylights out of me. The table was then raised about five feet off the ground , and the machine above me moved back and forth. A loud buzzing sound and there was no turning back; radiation was being administered. After the treatment, I returned to my locker, quickly slathered on lotion and went home.

Eventually, the burn worsened. In my case they used what is called a bolus, a rubbery pack that's approximately 8x10 inches. They would lay this on my burn and radiate it to bring the potency to the surface. They did this because the kind of cancer I had usually comes back in the skin. One day after a few weeks of treatment, the upper-left part of my back began to hurt. I looked in the mirror and noticed a large section of redness. I panicked, thinking that the radiation machine had gone wacko and overdosed me. The hospital staff reassured me that sometimes the burns can go all the way through your body. That information was not comforting!

My defiant attitude started to kick in when I decided to wait in my robe with neon flowers. I was no longer going to wear their shroudlike gowns. People loved the robe and started leaving me notes in the pockets.

My basement buddies became my support group as we watched TV shows together and commiserated. I made lifelong friendships in the waiting room. We had deep conversations about life and healing. We wiped each other's tears and reveled in each other's laughter. Although radiation felt like a full-time job and took my energy to the negative side of zero, I wouldn't give up what I learned about the human spirit. By the end of my treatments, my hair was sprouting. It was as soft as duckling fuzz. I gladly gave up my hat and turban.

My last day of radiation, I took a boom box in and dressed in black. Everyone seemed puzzled when I turned on "Back in Black" by AC/DC. This song is about having nine lives and escaping the noose; it seemed like an anthem to my survival. I had the whole place rockin. This selection of work you're about to read documents my experience through this phase of treatment. It gives a whole new meaning to the word "hot."

Right before radiation ended, the plan for maintenance care proceeded. It would involve a series of medications, the first of which was Tamoxifan. This daily pill would help deal with any estrogen left in my system. As another layer of protection, I was also put on monthly Lupron injections to induce chemical menopause. Because my tumor was estrogen receptor positive, these medications would reduce my chances of having a recurrence.

Not surprisingly, my thirty-four-year-old body didn't want to go into menopause and had become quite fond of estrogen. My ovaries rebelled by cramping and making several attempts to have a menstrual cycle. Finally, after a few months, they surrendered to the process. The changes in my body felt drastic and unpleasant. My mind was foggy and my moods were many.

This loss was further exacerbated by all of my friends who seemed to be able to have children with such ease. Going to baby showers or even seeing a baby made me ache. I felt guilty and angry all at the same time. I just wanted to understand *why* this devastating disease was ravaging not only my life but also my husband's and child's. I sunk into depression, and shockingly, doctors added more pills.

One day when Heidi (my photographer) came over for a photo shoot, she found me with pill bottles tied to my fingers with strings, like marionettes. We had a good laugh, and it helped her understand how I felt taking all those pills--like a puppet, controlled. The ever expanding pharmaceutical cupboard in my kitchen became a source of aggravation. I wanted Heidi to capture my relationship with these medications, and she certainly did!

You will see several examples in my writing in this section that reflect my love-hate relationship with treatment. I felt so much compassion for my body because it had to and has to continually process and respond to these medications. Now, because of the years of Lupron and other drugs, my bones are showing signs of deterioration, so, I'm taking osteoporosis medication once a month. On the love side, I have had years added to my life. I just celebrated my fortieth birthday, and my son is almost nine. I just need to let off some steam once in a while. Isn't complaining listed in the side effects? I often tell my husband that I want a trench coat to open up and reference with all the prescription printouts. That way I can prove that my behavior is induced by all the medications. Ha, ha! It just seems great to have an excuse for the range of moods, irritation and fatigue I experience.

BURN, BABY, BURN

Elevator doors screech
My instinct is to run

Basement corridors endless and cold
Something sinister happens here

I lie on a table made for science fiction
The plastic mold holds my pose
The machine hovers
Marks its targets
Beams its laser

Technicians escape behind thick walls
Program the doctor's recipe
Four to eight minutes
Cook until done

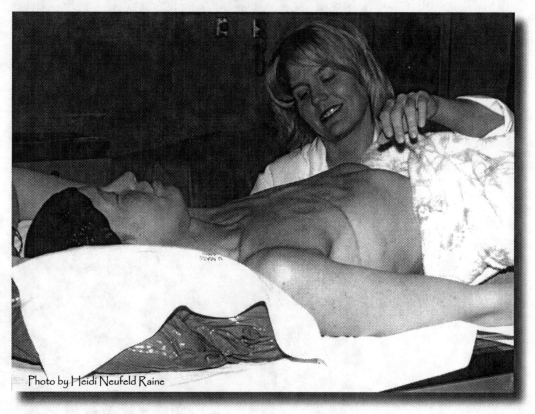

Photo by Heidi Neufeld Raine

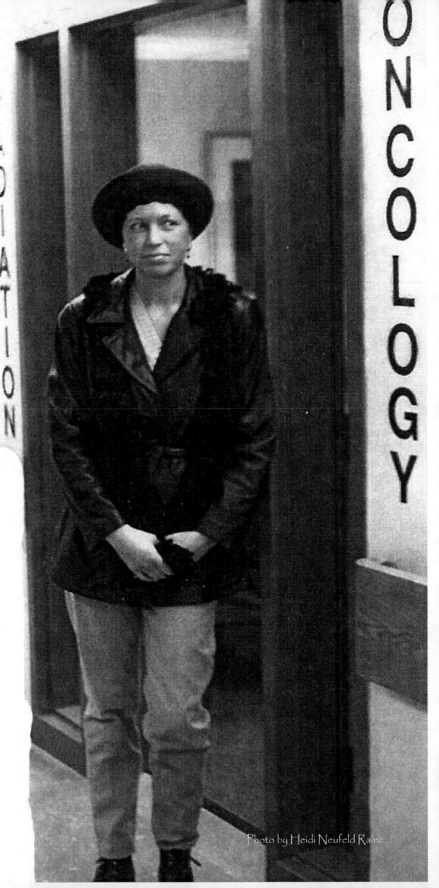

THE PRICE IS RIGHT

In the corner
A prehistoric Zenith
Television
Volume stuck on high
I change into my robe
Stuff clothes in a locker with
No combination

Victims of our pedigree
Our genetic mutations
We wait our turn
Count off the days
Burns on our skin
Bright evidence
Greasy lotion soothes

An old man changes the
Channel
The Price Is Right blares
And I smile
Oh no, the price is definitely
Too damn high

Photo by Heidi Neufeld Raine

HORRORMONES

I am officially manic
Time to check in to the Insanity Club Resort
Where walls are padded
Straight jackets handed out like robes

After the injection
I'll take the yellow rubber room
Where my screams can echo
As my ovaries choke

Tranquilize me
While my femininity slips away
So I won't notice the dullness of my hair
And parched skin

I feel flushed in more ways than one
Hot flashes repeat themselves
Chemical menopause isn't for sissies
I didn't know neurons could play tag

My thoughts run away like unruly children
My brain a playground

I could explode with frustration
My body tries to understand why it can't bleed
Detonate me please

NURSE'S COMMUNION

Jaundice-yellow containers
White, dusty pills
Sacrament on my eager tongue
Bitter and gritty

Tepid wine relieves my mouth
I need the euphoria
Like the devil needs sin

In twenty minutes
Thoughts soften
No longer tearing and jagged
Blessed numbness reigns

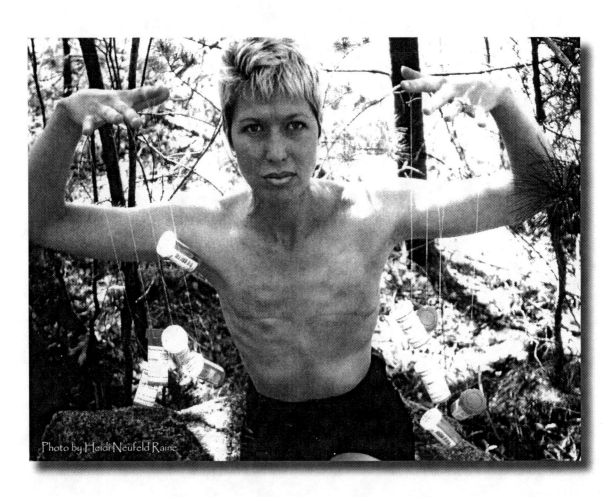

Photo by Heidi Neufeld Raine

LOOPRON
My version of "Twist and Shout"

Here we go!
Shake it up, baby
Twist the medication and shout
Come on, come on, baby
Stick your backside out

Shake it, shake it up, baby
I'm gonna scream and pout
The three inch needles going in no doubt

You know I run, little girl
I run so fine
Take that needle out, don't take your time

You know it makes me crazy
Makes me sweat
I can't wait 'til it's over
I wanna drive off in my Corvette!

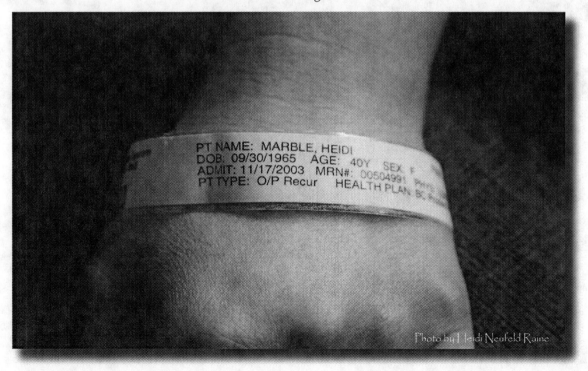

Photo by Heidi Neufeld Raine

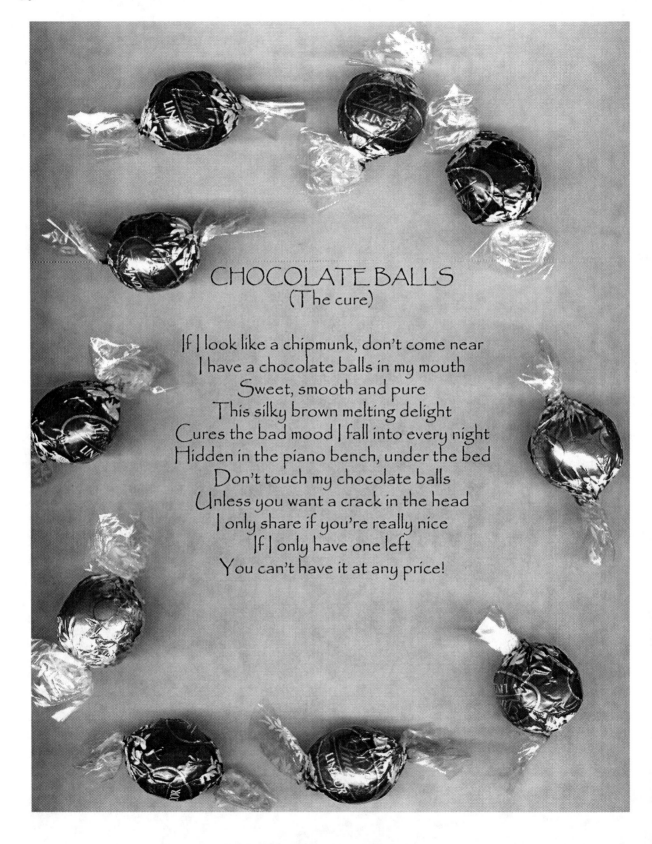

CHOCOLATE BALLS
(The cure)

If I look like a chipmunk, don't come near
I have a chocolate balls in my mouth
Sweet, smooth and pure
This silky brown melting delight
Cures the bad mood I fall into every night
Hidden in the piano bench, under the bed
Don't touch my chocolate balls
Unless you want a crack in the head
I only share if you're really nice
If I only have one left
You can't have it at any price!

Part Four
Coping
and
Recovery

This section of poems is born from the variety of emotions I felt after active treatment stopped. I was frightened, yet hopeful, about my future. Six months after my radiation therapy ended, my husband finished his supervision of Boston's cable stay bridge. It was time for us to move on to another bridge in another state. In many ways, this was a new start, but we left behind deep and powerful friendships. When we first moved to California, we rented a beautiful home from Dave and Denise Fisher. He is a doctor and she is a cancer survivor with a wonderful attitude.

Denise and I quickly built a friendship, and we started training for a three-day breast cancer walk. A few months later, with our $150 walking shoes, we were ready to go. We walked thirteen miles until we collapsed under a tree questioning ourselves. After a few more hours and a lot of moaning and groaning, we made it to our base camp. It was somewhat of a surprise that the camp was set up in the middle of a horse track. The night was long as we listened to port-a-potty doors slamming.

At the crack of dawn, there was an announcement over the loudspeaker and before we knew it, jockeys were running their horses around the track. I called Troy on my cell phone and said "come and get me!" Denise, however, carried on and finished the walk. She lost her toenails but kept her pride.

My body was not the same after treatment. My blood counts remained low and I suffered from bouts of fatigue. I came down with lymphedema, or swelling of the arm from the removal of the lymph nodes. I had to use compression bandages to control the swelling in addition to going to rehabilitation. I also had to come to grips with the emotional toll cancer had taken. There were times I felt so strong and sure. Then in a heartbeat, I would sink into fear and trepidation. I had nightmares and terrors about my cancer returning. I always had plenty of food in the house and bought Blake his clothes months in advance, just in case. The what- ifs took over my thinking.

My challenge was to rebuild my life, my body and my spirit. I soon realized that healing is as unique as the snowflakes that fall. Each person heals in his or her own time. At my core, I felt confused; I started searching for who I was supposed to become. I often felt like a little child lacking independence. I was angry and tired of being sick and giving things up to cancer.

Hopefully, my upcoming hysterectomy will be my final physical sacrifice. I am no longer willing to drag cancer around like a ball and chain. Dealing with the fear of recurrence is getting easier as each year passes. Still, there is a steady disturbance that I can't seem to eradicate. It helps me to be "sassy" towards cancer. I often tell cancer how much I despise its existence. I am choosing health and life. Cancer picked the wrong girl to mess with!

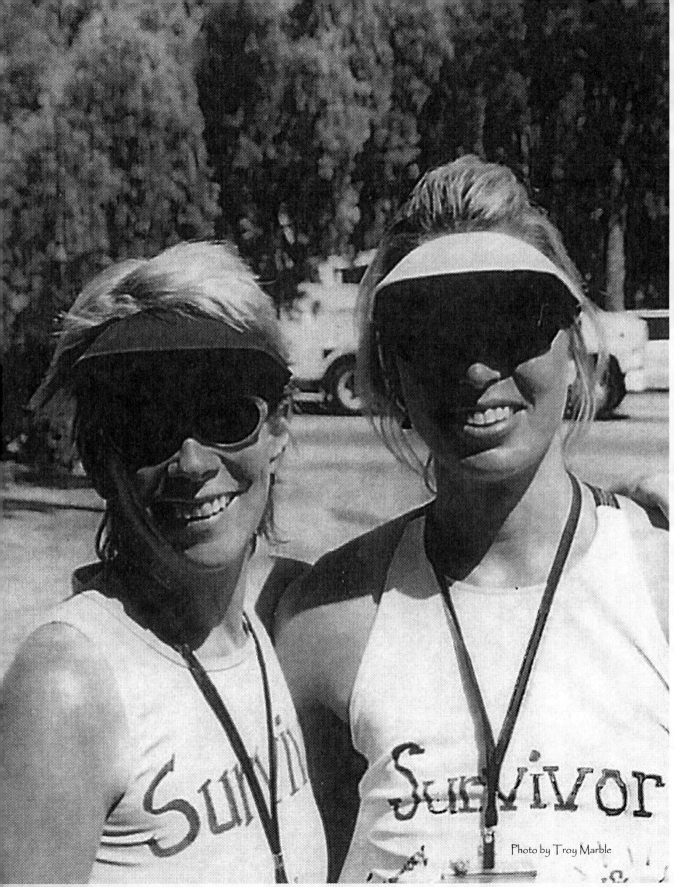

Photo by Troy Marble

BOOMERANG
Regarding my fear of recurrence

Down under in this barren land
You are shaped to return
No matter how hard you are thrown
I don't want you to come back
Like a nasty weed
I don't want to be the soil you choose
Your seeds and roots are not welcome
I will remain desolate

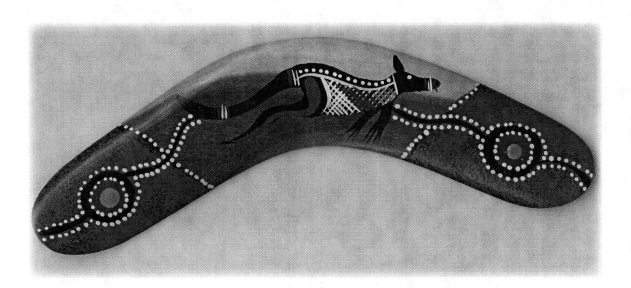

THIEF

I should have bolted the door
Hidden the key
Heard the alarms
No one saw you
Master of disguise
Hands in gloves
Knife at my throat
You took my breasts
My hair
My womb
Pawned my libido for pocket change
Did they catch you?
When will we know?
I want to be left alone
There is nothing else to take

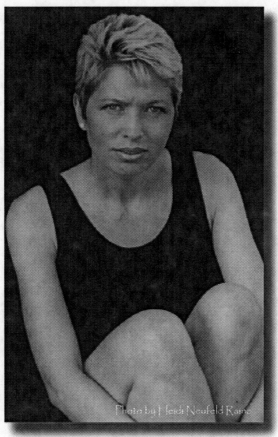

Photo by Heidi Neufeld Raine

YELLOW CENTER

This poem is about the little girl inside me who is so vulnerable.
During the course of my illness, I often felt like a child.

I see you hiding behind bleached eyes
You tremble and hug your pain
Between wet sheets you cry
Twist your caramel hair around your finger
The night is blank and long
The breakfast table waits
You pierce the yellow center of the egg
Taste its fertile yolk
The crisp bacon savored
I smell the rubbed leather of your boots
You go to your well-groomed horses
Find refuge in their large wet eyes

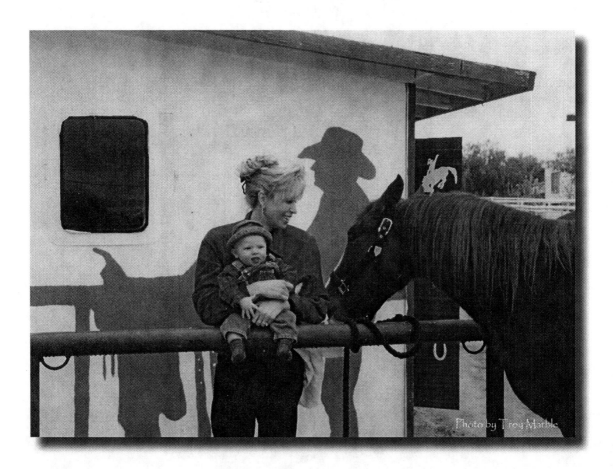

Photo by Troy Marble

I'M ALIVE

I know the infirmary
The bulging medical file
My abbreviated name
My case number

I'm ALIVE

I hear the guesswork
The phantom hovers
I understand trepidation

I'm ALIVE!

Inside this cracked shell
There is a soul
Iridescent with no parameters
My essence still remains

I'm ALIVE!!!!

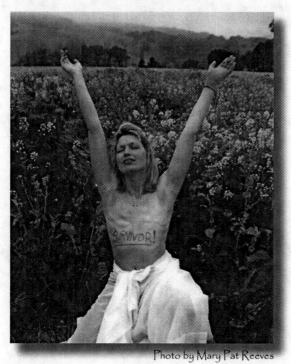

Photo by Mary Pat Reeves

LYMPHE SCREAMA

My arm deformed
Heavy and uncooperative
The ruby glass I hold shatters
I put oil under my rings
I twist and pull
My fingers full of stagnant fluid
Posed with my hand above my heart
I struggle with the compression bandages
My fingernails turn blue
I can't pick up my son
Can't carry groceries
I wish the lymphatic fluid would flow
Clearly and freely

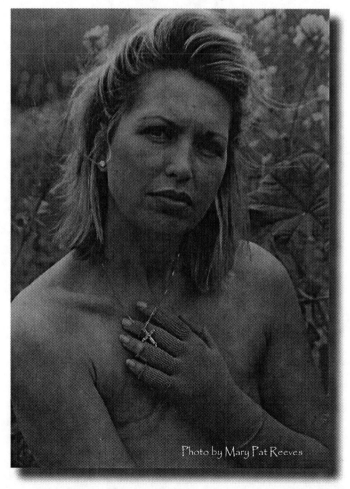

Photo by Mary Pat Reeves

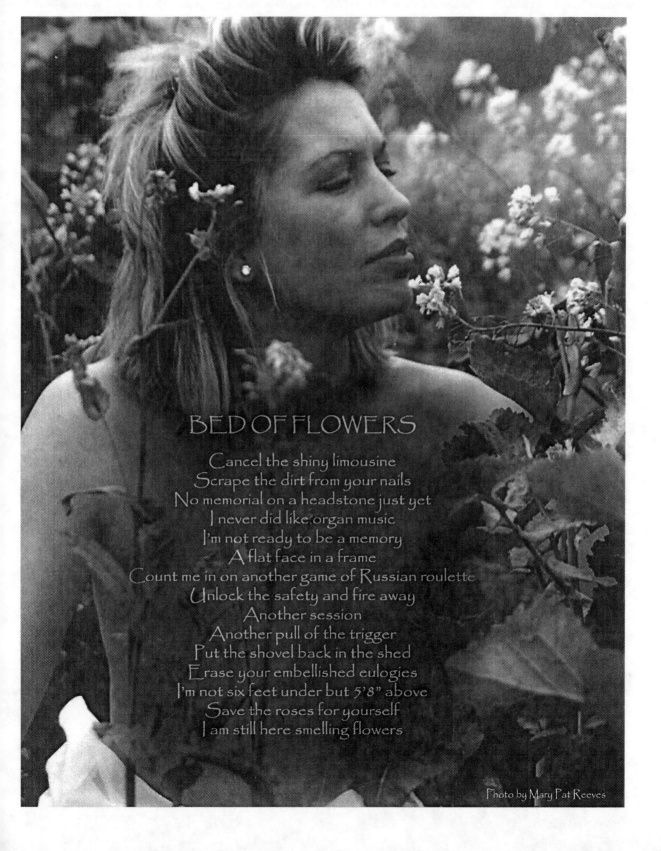

BED OF FLOWERS

Cancel the shiny limousine
Scrape the dirt from your nails
No memorial on a headstone just yet
I never did like organ music
I'm not ready to be a memory
A flat face in a frame
Count me in on another game of Russian roulette
Unlock the safety and fire away
Another session
Another pull of the trigger
Put the shovel back in the shed
Erase your embellished eulogies
I'm not six feet under but 5'8" above
Save the roses for yourself
I am still here smelling flowers

Photo by Mary Pat Reeves

INTERNAL CLOTHING

Thick needles rest in my seams
The mending has become overwhelming
So much is torn and tattered
I am a spool unwinding
I suck my bloody finger
Carefully tie knots so I don't slip through the eye of my existence
I tear so easily
Dull scissors can't cut a straight line around the brittle pattern I wear
I am a collection of assorted remnants
Worn thin

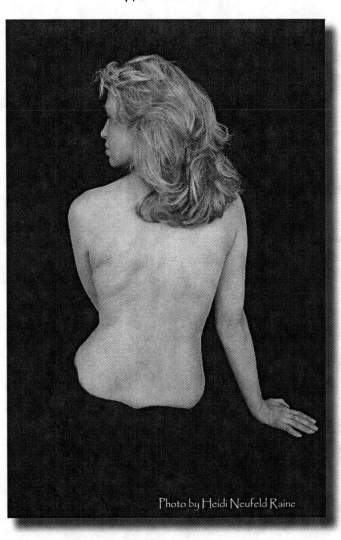

Photo by Heidi Neufeld Raine

LUGGAGE

I climb the stairs to the attic
My suitcases wait
Dirty, empty
I clean the evidence of stillness away
Reveal their scars
I find some beach sand from days past
Rub it into the palm of my hand

I decide we have more places to explore
We will be together until we reach our final destination
Too tired to hold our contents anymore

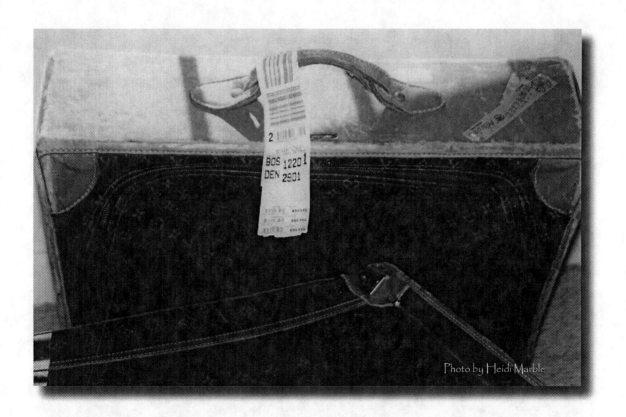

Photo by Heidi Marble

OLD AND GRAY

I hope we can live until we are old and gray
Rocking and eating the day away
Golfing for you
Shopping for me
Spoiling our grandkids on a charging spree
Long lazy mornings
Beach days in the sun
Our wrinkled hands becoming one
Memories reflected back in our eyes
You accepting the cellulite on my thighs
Me rubbing your shiny bald head
Maybe I'll even have my hair dyed red!
May we pass to the next life lying side by side
Saying, "I love you honey, it's been a great ride"

Troy's and my collection of old-people figurines

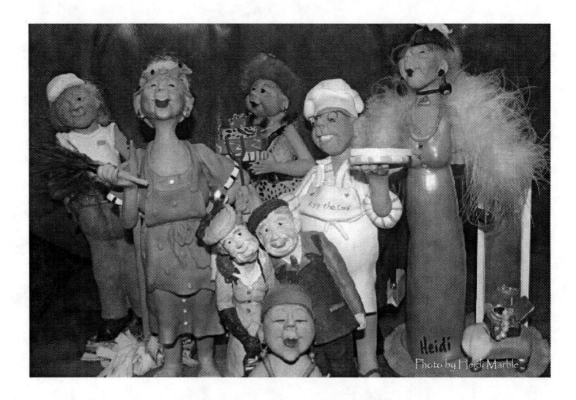

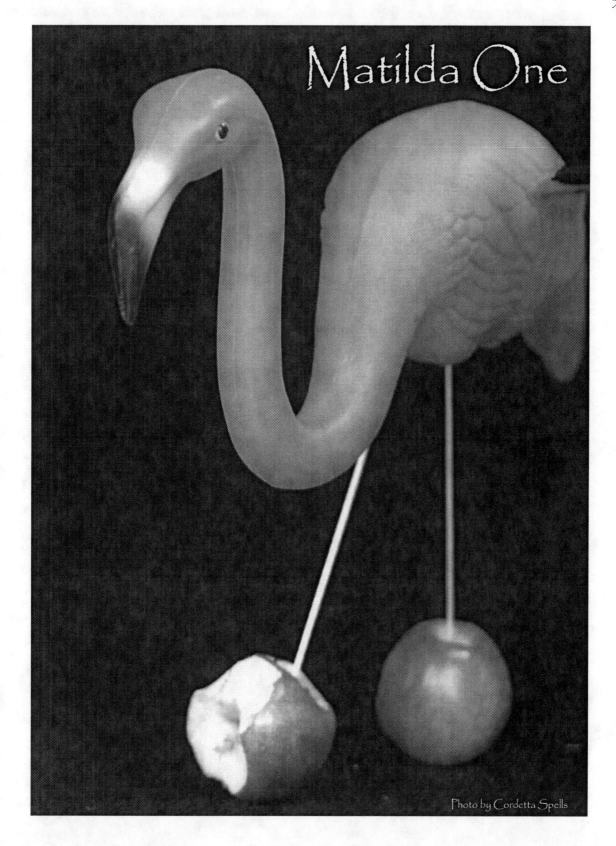

Matilda One

Photo by Cordetta Spells

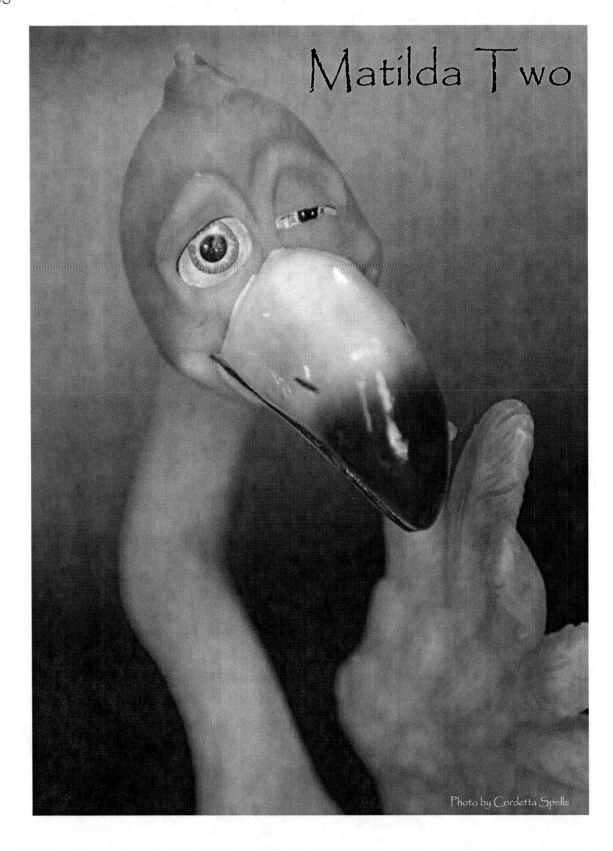

Matilda Two

Photo by Cordetta Spells

MATILDA

It is often difficult to excavate humor when dealing with a crisis in life. Not only did I find humor, but I also found deep friendship with Kimberly and Yasemin. We connected at a support group for cancer patients at Beth Israel Deaconess Hospital in Boston. Our relationship spread out into nourishing rituals like eating at my neighbor's Italian cafe and going to Hope Lodge. Hope Lodge is a charming Victorian home nestled in Worchester, Massachusetts. Its sole purpose is to support and house people coming from other states or countries to receive treatment. They held a monthly support group in the living room. It was such a safe, welcoming place to embrace the difficult issues cancer brings.

During one of our monthly get-togethers, I introduced the idea of having a humorous object that we could rotate during times of need. Since plastic pink flamingos were on sale, two for $5.99, and are bullet proof, we decided that a flamingo would work. Then came the arduous job of naming the flamingo: "Matilda" somehow emerged as appropriate.

One could never tell where and when Matilda might show up. Luckily, we have never been reported to a bird rescue program. Matilda has experienced abuse both verbal and physical. Not only have we made fun of her vibrant color and out-of-proportion body, but we have also replaced her legs with margarita spoons.

When I moved from New England to Northern California, Yasemin and Kimberly put Matilda in my front yard the night before I left for California. The poor bird has been mailed back and forth at least a dozen times. She has also been misplaced on several occasions. I have often wondered if this was intentional.

As my beautiful friend Kimberly began to deal with the return of her cancer, I felt it was only appropriate that Matilda should go back to her. I flew to Boston, and Kimberly and I went to our Italian cafe. When the time was right, I placed Matilda on the table. Kimberly's laughter filled the restaurant until everyone was laughing with us. She couldn't get over the fact that I carried our bird on the plane for seven hours before sneaking her into the restaurant.

Matilda is now proudly displayed in Kimberly and Paul's living room for all their guests to enjoy. When she heard I wanted to put a picture of Matilda in this book, she seemed very anxious to ship her back. I insisted that Matilda's body double would suffice.

My photographer Cordetta invited me to see Matilda's photo-shoot preparation. Much to my dismay, Matilda had kebob skewers for legs with two half-eaten apples to hold her upright. Once again, Matilda brought unexpected laughter.

NO MORE SHACKLES

No jury, judge or appeal
I will not be sentenced to food on plastic trays
Hard mattresses or solitary confinement
You will not have to visit me through a glass wall
No longer on death row
Untie the noose
It won't be on my neck
I am planning my escape
While cancer's suggestion smashes my face into the wall
Unlock the ball and chain I've been dragging
I've paid my bail, done my time
No flashing lights or backseat rides
I'm driving now
Faith as my partner
Hope as my weapon
When I am old and gray
I will die without shackles
Leaving my stamped clothes behind

Photo by Cordetta Spells

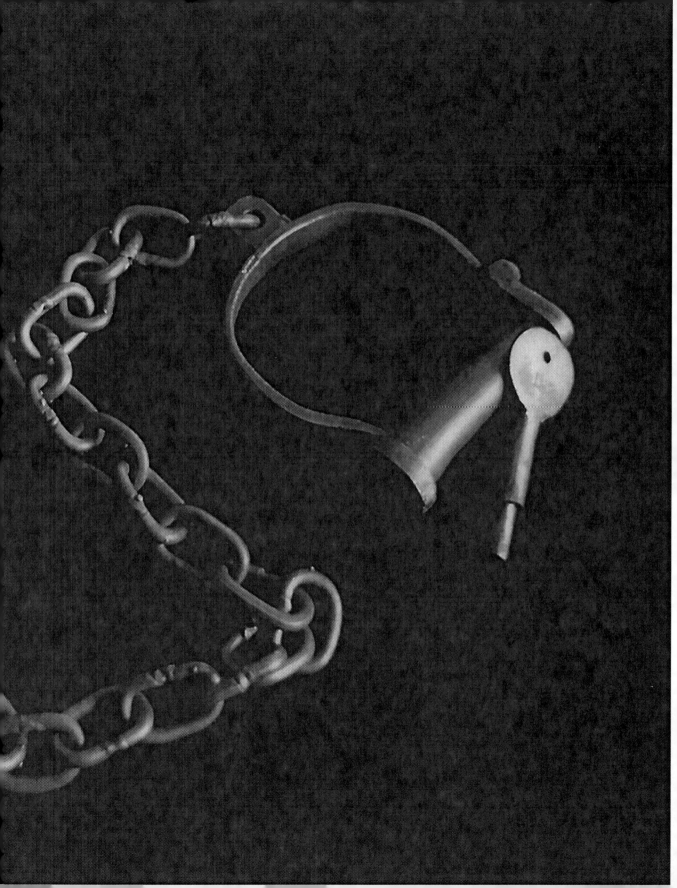

BIRDS FOR SALE

In my mid twenties
I lick away at my chocolate ice cream
The mall a haven for shoppers
Puppies in the window
Wood chips on their new fur
Price tags too high for my crinkled-up ten-dollar bill
I wander past the silvery fish
In their bubbling tanks
Then I hear the frantic thumping
Of newly captured birds hitting the glass
Blood is wet and smeared
Their beaks bleed
They repeat their fruitless escape
The clerk sees my horror
Shrugs me off with
"They get used to it"
I want to buy them all
Set them free into the blue sky
Now
On the tail end of thirty-nine
I hear the frantic thumping of my heart
A glass wall between me and everything I hope for
Afraid to fly

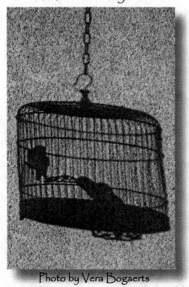

Photo by Vera Bogaerts

FULL PRICE
Regarding my upcoming hysterectomy

Cancer, I've put you on clearance
On some crowded rack in the back of my mind
I don't want to wear you anymore
No more catwalks to show your latest designs
Backstage I strip bare
The doctor tells me we need to cut and sew
You fancy my uterus and ovaries
For your spring collection of medical couture
I'll remove my polish
Scrub my face clean
Lay my body down for your alterations
Under the harsh, white lights
No negotiation
I'll pay full price

Photo by Cordetta Spells

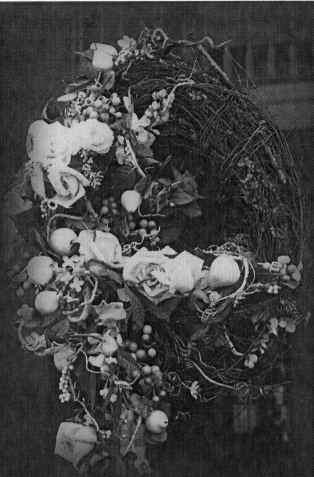

Part Five
Miracles
and
Faith

Photo by Heidi Neufeld Raine

After my double mastectomy and removal of eighteen lymph nodes, we waited for the pathology report that would forecast the next attempt to save my life. It was understood ahead of time that it wasn't a matter of *if* the cancer was in the lymph nodes but in how many? However, you'll see that I prayed for a miracle, for no node involvement and for life. During the waiting period, a sparrow couple created a beautiful nest in a wreath that hung on the screen of my front door. Every morning, I would drag myself downstairs, open the door and watch them work away. Luckily for me, they weren't afraid, even though they could probably feel my breath. The only thing between me and them was a thin layer of screen.

Soon, four blue eggs rested inside this amazing cup of safety they created. I watched as these new parents took turns tending to the eggs. They even let me take pictures. Then, the day my surgeon was supposed to call with my results, I heard all kinds of bird commotion. I opened the door and saw that all four eggs had hatched. The chicks were chirping and had their mouths open big and wide. Friends and family commented that the chicks' being born was a sign from God.

At 5:37 Dr. Troyan called with pure joy in her voice. She told me that not one lymph node had cancer and that the breast tissue had mostly dead cells. The tumor had clear margins (no cancer left behind), it seemed we finally had the upper hand. This was the best possible news. The fight wasn't over yet, but the tide had definitely started to turn. Instead of planning for my death, I started to plan for survival. My first goal was to watch my son start kindergarten.

When I went to put my wreath away the following winter, I took the abandoned nest and framed it. The following spring, I hung the wreath again; this time I included some of the hair I had lost. Before I knew it, the sparrows showed up and weaved the most beautiful nest with my hair. In a few days, they laid four more blue eggs, which hatched on the first anniversary of my diagnosis. We moved to San Francisco; I hung my wreath; and guess what! More sparrows, and four more blue eggs! Of course they hatched on the day of my second anniversary!

As you will see in this section, these signs from God were essential for me to maintain my will to survive. Although I questioned and struggled with faith, I knew at the deepest level that God loved me. I seemed stuck in wondering what I did or didn't do to have this disease in my life. Enjoy the pictures of the nests, take notice of the one with blonde strands of hair. So many days I wanted to crawl in a giant nest under soft breast feathers and rest in safety.

Probably the most amazing experience I had with the birds' nest was during an afternoon session of rehabilitation exercises. I had gone up to my room, and my arm was hurting from radiation and lymph node removal. I had a hand-out of assigned exercises, so I lay down on my bed to stretch. I decided to position myself sideways. The night before I had read about a religion that believes God resides at the head of a sick person's bed. I wondered if He was at the head of my bed. Suddenly, my eyes were drawn to a plaque I'd had for years that was above the headboard. In the middle of this plaque was a birds' nest with four blue eggs just like the one I had been given at my front door. At that moment, I knew I was going to live.

Also, you will notice a silver cross around my neck in one of the pictures. After my father died from emphysema at age fifty-nine, I asked for his cross. All my life, he wore it around his neck; he never took it off. The back side of the cross is worn from his moving and breathing. My dad was a cowboy, a cop and Dirty Harry's twin.

When we would ride horses into the desert sunset, I would always notice the cross shining inside his slightly unbuttoned shirt. When he worked outside in the desert sun, the cross would drip with his sweat. He never verbalized what it meant to him, but I knew it was important. The day he died, I walked out of the hospital with the cross in the palm of my hand. It has been with me through thick and thin as a representation of faith and sacrifice. The poem about my dad and his cross was written years ago, but I feel it connects with my faith today.

The cross, nests and prayers became my clarity when everything seemed hopeless. Throughout my journey, even now, I receive affirmation that God and His angels have my back. My survival is considered a miracle, and I am thankful to be alive.

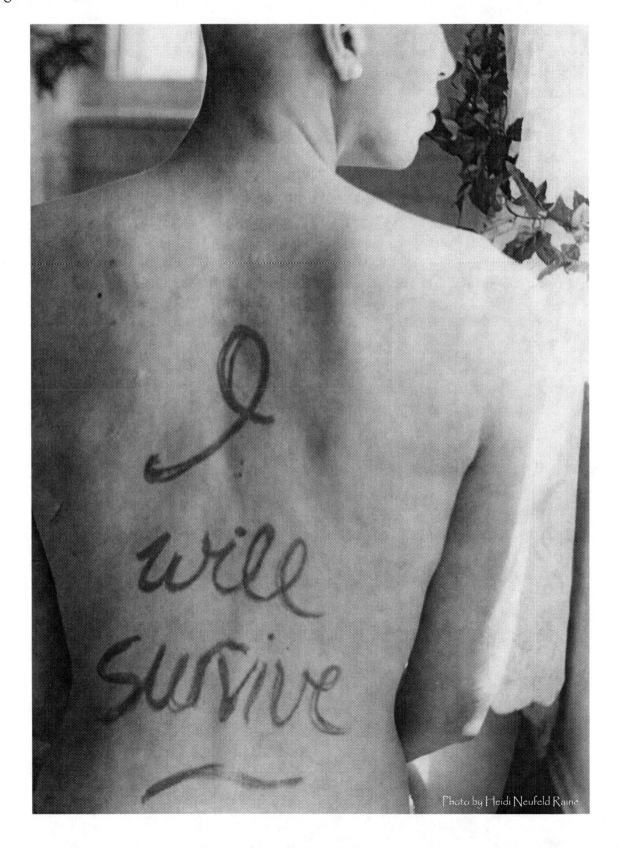

Photo by Heidi Neufeld Raine

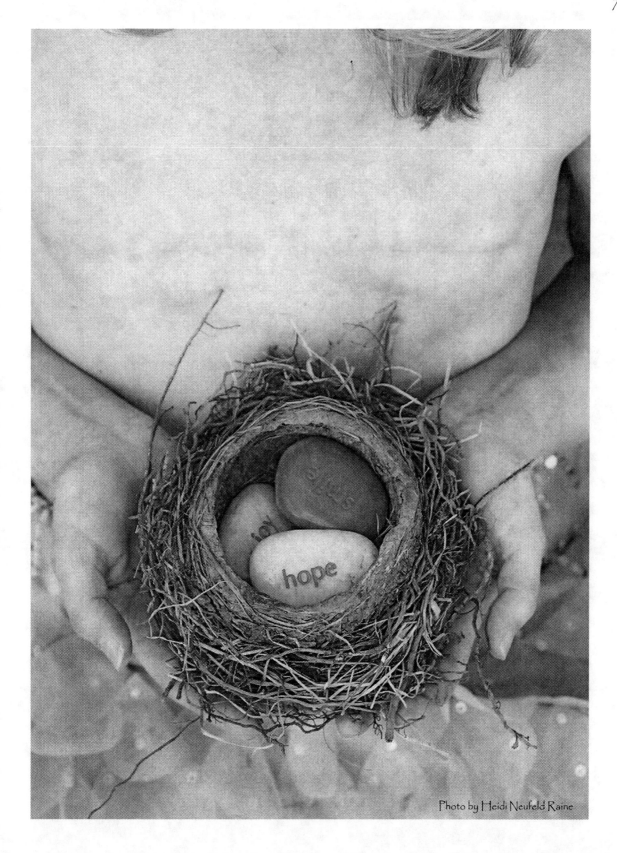

Photo by Heidi Neufeld Raine

DREAM WEAVERS

She wove her nest at my door
Amidst flowers
Soon four eggs lay there
Speckled and blue

I wanted to crawl under her warmth
Protected in her feathers
Kept safe in her circle of branches
Lulled by her song
Would I ever push through my shell?
Stretch my fragile wings?

The day her eggs hatched
My cancer was gone

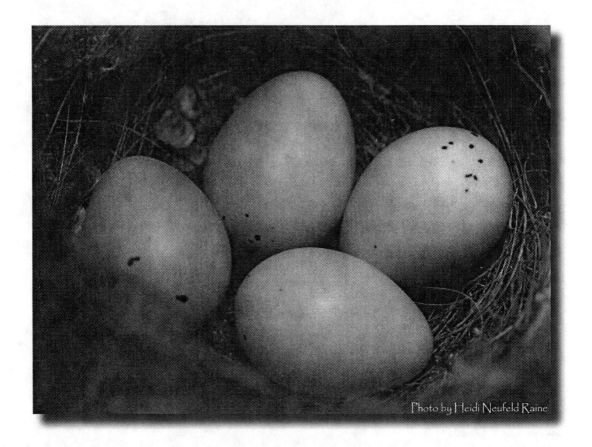

Photo by Heidi Neufeld Raine

POINT OF VIEW

Starved of hope
I rest on sheets of faded roses
My four poster bed my new home
Contort my arm into assigned stretches
Hiss at the world
Every part hurts
Tears strain from my eyes
Torturous rehabilitation

I don't know what to believe
Does God really reside at the head of a sick person's bed?
He must be holding someone else in His lap
I notice the plaque above the headboard
Its center a nest with four blue eggs
Just like the ones laid at my door
Rebirth

Photo by Heidi Marble

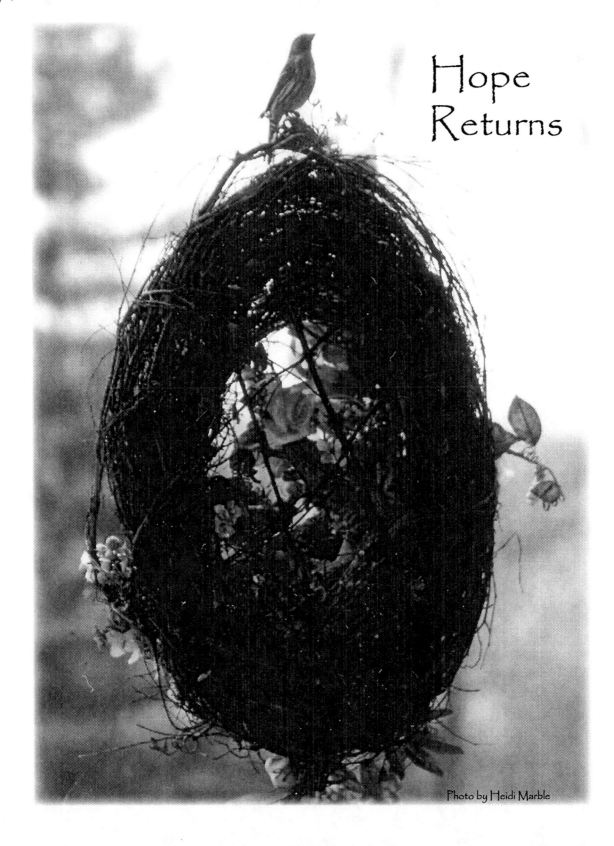

Hope Returns

Photo by Heidi Marble

MY FATHER, ART THOU IN HEAVEN?

My Father, art Thou in heaven?
Do You hear my name?

My cup runs over
Yet my thirst is great

Will You deliver me from this suffering?
If my will be done
I want earth instead of heaven

In the valley of the shadow of death
I fear the evil
As cancer trespasses against me

I search for green pastures
Still waters to restore my soul

I want goodness and mercy
All the days of my life

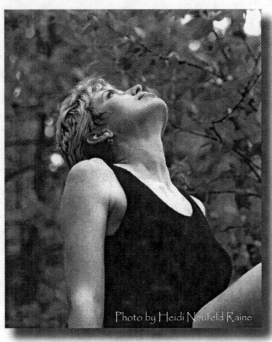

Photo by Heidi Neufeld Raine

DADDY'S CROSS

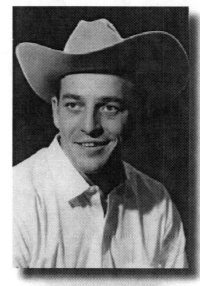

What happened to my cowboy, Daddy?
Remember we used to ride
Me on the pony
You on the black stallion
The sound of your lighter
Your brilliant cigarette
Weekend rodeos
Bulls and bucking broncos
Your suede chaps and silver spurs
Blankets and saddles
Country music in your white pickup
I still remember your cross glistening on your chest
Your sweat dripping while you lifted hay
You taught me about taking the upper hand
Not showing fear
Riding until you could no longer hold on
Then mounting again until the horse understood
That you meant business
Cancer is the beast I've tamed
I've learned to bridle my power
Dust myself off
Not go down without a fight
When I pray
Your cross's chain spills into the palm of my hand
I fold my fingers around all I have left of you

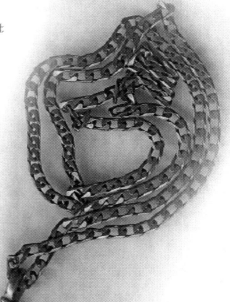

LET'S MAKE A DEAL

In this sanctuary
My dad's silver cross around my neck
Familiar hymns resonate
The stained glass changes with the sky's disposition
My Bible is worn
I kneel on calloused knees
At the foot of the cross
And beg for salvation
Holy water still wet on my forehead
I bargain for more time

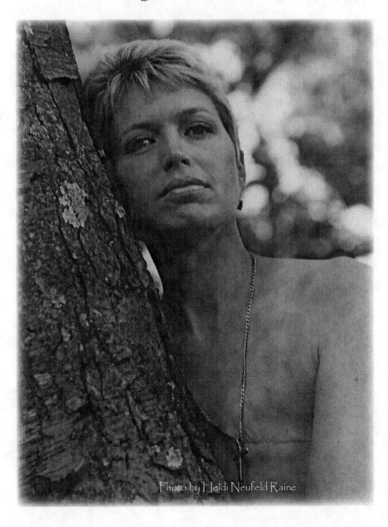

Photo by Heidi Neufeld Raine

Part Six
Family
and
Friends

Photo by Heidi Neufeld Raine

This section contains poems written in celebration of family and friends who have stayed by my side as I have fought cancer.

Troy is the love of my life. I met him when I was the tender age of fifteen. He was eighteen at the time. It was love at first sight for me; he didn't even know I existed. Then one night, during the last song of a spring dance, he asked me to dance with him. We dated through the summer and I fell deeply in love with him. He broke my heart when he went away to college. Our paths took us in different directions. Nonetheless, I always thought of Troy and compared him to every man I dated. Three years later, while I was in college, Troy's younger brother was in a car accident. Roger and I had remained friends, since we were the same age. Roger called from the emergency room and asked me to go be with him. Much to my surprise, Troy was there. I thought he was still going to a college four hours north. Well, Roger recovered, and Troy and I started to date. Ten months later Troy and I were married.

I never thought when we said our vows that cold winter night in the mountains of Arizona that cancer would be in our future. He has loved me no matter what I looked or felt like. The most profound testimony to our bond was during the worst part of my chemotherapy treatment. I retreated to my bedroom after dinner; I was feeling dizzy and unsettled. I thought having a warm bath might help. I undressed and crumpled to the floor. My body could no longer stay upright. I lay naked, cold and curled up on the hard tile. I attempted to drag myself to the open door so I could shut it. I simply didn't have the strength. I pulled into a ball and wept silently, afraid someone would find me. My worst fears were realized when I heard footsteps coming closer. I prayed that it wasn't my son.

Then I felt Troy's strong, warm hand on my back. Without a word he shut the door and ran the bath water. He lifted me into the bathtub. I have never loved anyone more that I loved him at that moment. Up to that point, I had concealed my wounds and weight loss. His touch made me feel connected. I could feel his love and acceptance. I realized he loved my spirit as much or more than my body. During our twenty years of marriage, he has loved me to levels I didn't know existed.

Blake is my miracle boy. After struggling with years of infertility, I finally conceived my beautiful baby. He was born on his due date, a whopping nine pounds three ounces, with loads of blond curly hair. Troy and I have been so amazed by Blake's spirit and love of life. He bounds with energy and talent. His heart is bright and it illuminates our lives in so many ways. Watching him grow is like watching the sunrise every day. He takes the darkness and fills it with color and energy. We can't wait to see how his life unfolds. Our love for him is so intense and complete.

My mom, Joy, was meant to be my mother. She adopted me while I was still in the womb. She has loved me and has been a constant source of strength my whole life. Our lives were destined to connect. Her love has prepared me for all the ups and downs of life. We talk everyday. She is still my compass; her wisdom is my oxygen.

My beautiful grandma (aka Wongee, a name I gave her before I had a phonics lesson) is my mom's mom and had lost the love of her life to a heart attack nine months before I was born. From the moment we laid eyes on each other, a special relationship was in place. Her home was a place of joy and filled with grandma things. She let my brother and me jump from bed to bed and let us eat too many cookies; she never told on us when we were naughty. There were late-night trips to Dairy Queen to get Dilly Bars on those blistering summer nights. She would lay a towel in the backseat of her Buick to catch melting ice cream and then she'd let us run through the sprinklers in her backyard to get clean. We made mud pies that she claimed were delicious. Her love for us has been deep and loyal. She is fading, but she will always be my Wongee.

My brother Justin Jon came into my life when I was seven. I was resentful of his presence because he wasn't a girl. Also, he took all the attention away from me. For this he paid dearly until he was thirteen. In spite of my big-sister antics, he always tolerated me. His kindness was evident at a very young age. In 2004, when he was only thirty-two, we lost him to pneumonia without so much as a warning. I miss him beyond explanation.

Kimberly and Yasemin are featured in this section. They became my fellow warriors during my illness. Kimberly has the most beautiful voice and laugh, not to mention the courage of a lion. After three rounds with cancer, she still retains her grace and faith. Her advice and friendship have carved hope into my spirit. Yasemin has the most dazzling green eyes and infectious smile. We have had so much fun together over the years. Our healing retreat in New Hampshire felt like a teenage girls' sleepover. We talked and laughed until the wee hours of the morning. Kimberly and Yasemin have been there with me every step of the way. I will love both of them forever.

Kathleen, Rachel and Susan were not only my neighbors but my lifeline. Fate had placed a social worker (Kathleen), a spiritual guide (Rachel) and a nurse (Susan) in the houses that surrounded mine. They cooked for me, watched my son and took me outside when I was isolating myself. They cried, laughed and went through this experience with me. We spent four years in each other's company, and I learned so much from these angelic women. Without them I would have been lost. They lent me their strength, without flinching; they fully supported our family. I can never begin to explain the difference they made in my survival.

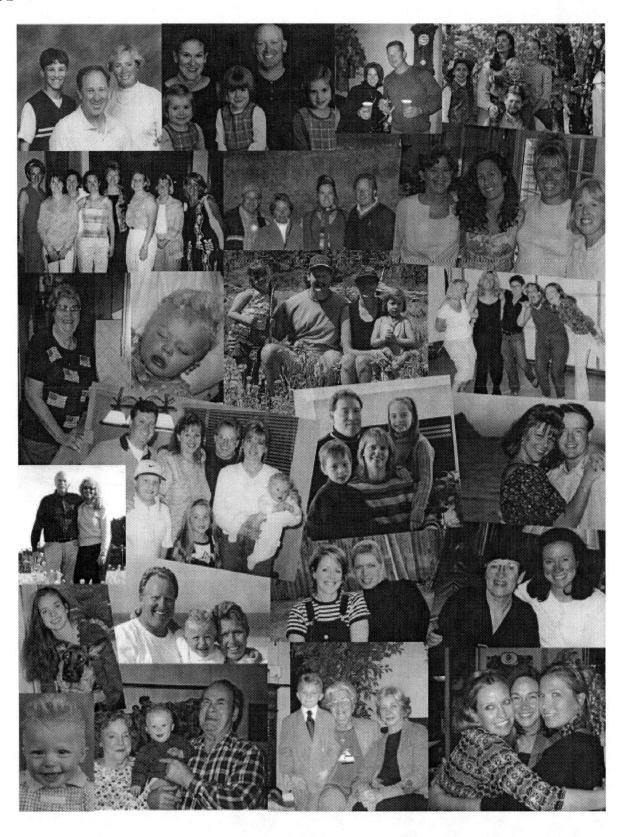

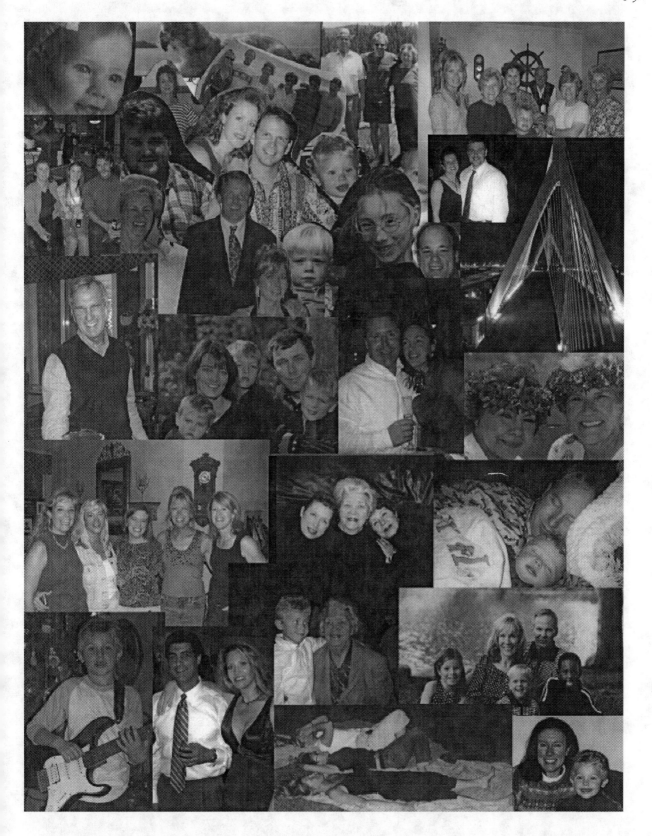

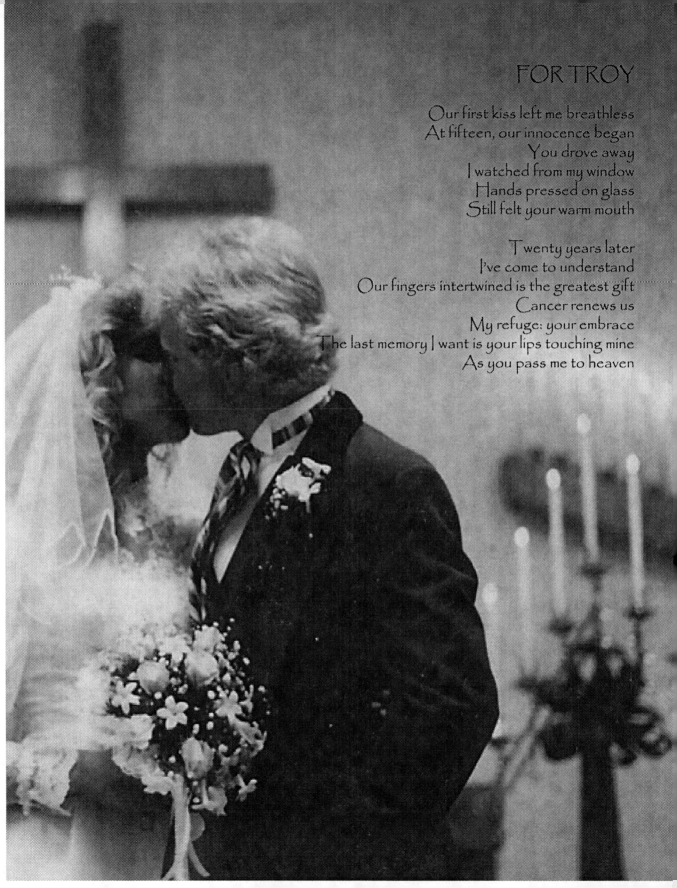

FOR TROY

Our first kiss left me breathless
At fifteen, our innocence began
You drove away
I watched from my window
Hands pressed on glass
Still felt your warm mouth

Twenty years later
I've come to understand
Our fingers intertwined is the greatest gift
Cancer renews us
My refuge: your embrace
The last memory I want is your lips touching mine
As you pass me to heaven

WHAT WILL I LEAVE YOU?
For Troy

Rock me like a child
In your arms
Protect me a little longer
Say you understand
Tolerate my wounds
I know I slow you down
It makes me ache
What will happen to us?
What will I leave you?
Will my life have been enough?
Feel the courage in my sadness
Strength in my rage
We are not the same as before
Pull me back in
Your love heals me

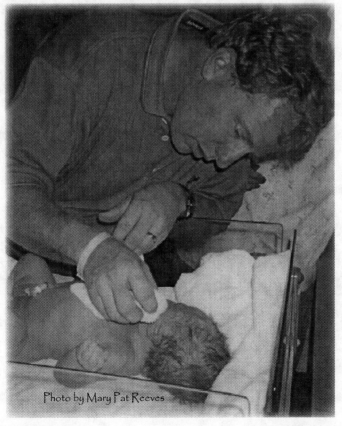

Photo by Mary Pat Reeves

SWEET ATTENTION

The light is never absent
It just moves in and out of darkness
Frozen dialogue begins to thaw
Dark ink bleeds onto thin white paper
I feel your touch
I drink your attention
Frenzied lapping of every last drop
Your mouth presses on mine
Coarse whiskers
I furrow my brow
Your hands hold memories
Of a body I'll never have again
Grief is in your fingertips

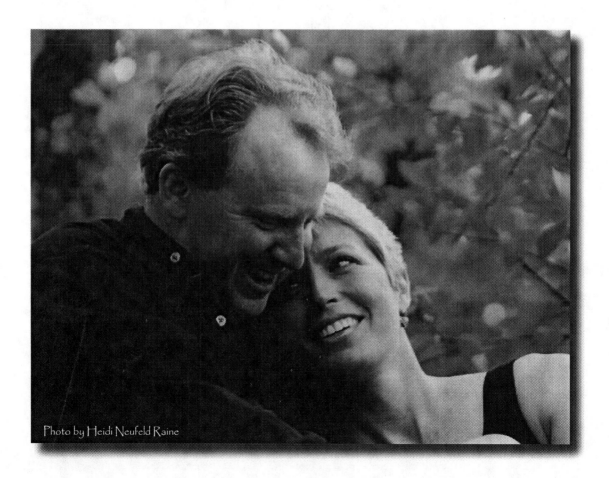

Photo by Heidi Neufeld Raine

MY SON

Flesh of my flesh
Your skin gives me a reason to fight
My eyes in yours
Strands of blue and green

The day you were born
I was introduced to miracles
My milk spilled for you
Primitive comfort

I want to get lost in those days again
Your restless hand brought to peace in mine
Feeling the delicate pull of your breath

This broken body needs to see you shed me like skin
I won't give up until
My hand can rest in the strength of yours

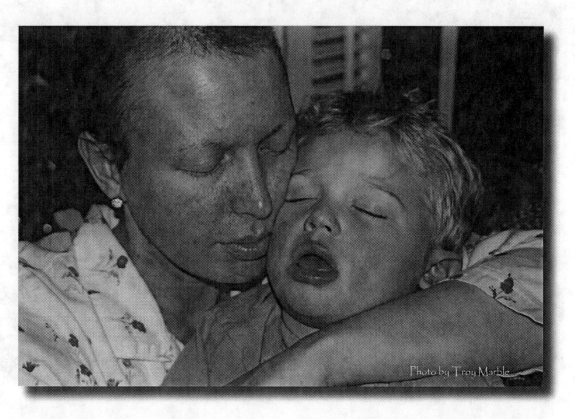

Photo by Troy Marble

WATERFALL BLUE

Inspired by seeing my six-year-old son sleeping with his dog, Angel

Waterfall blue melts the darkness
Stars extinguished by the morning's breath
A milky curtain floats into stillness
I notice the rain-stained window
Your blankets bundled around you
Your perfect mouth slightly open
My heart collides into love
You are my son
Can I keep you forever in this warm place?
The sun igniting your golden hair
Your dog curled at your feet
Your sleep so pure
I am afraid to move
To disturb this moment

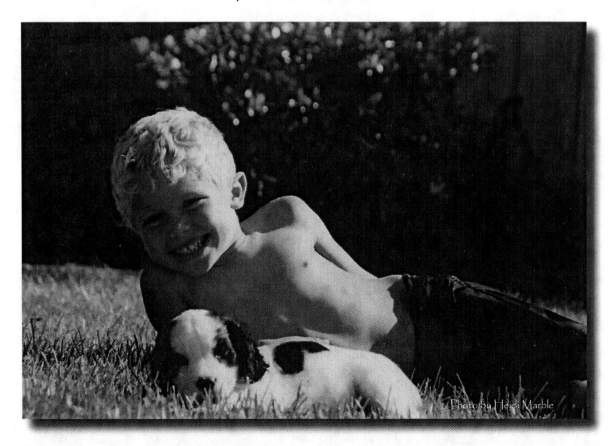

Photo by Heidi Marble

MEANT TO BE MY MOTHER

A September desert morning 1965
The watercolor sunrise washes away the darkness
I take my first breath with the sting of a slap
She was too young
You were there to take me home
Waiting so long in your emptiness
For a child
You fed my hunger
Swaddled me in handmade quilts
Placed my ear to your heart
I heard your love
You were meant to be my mother
Raising me from baby to woman
I was too young
Cancer came
I waited in my emptiness for your arrival
Thousands of miles you traveled
To run my home
Feed my hunger
Swaddle my son
Place his ear to your heart
After thirty-four years
You nourished and bathed my body again
You saved me twice

Photo by Mary Pat Reeves

WOO, HOO, HOO, HOO
About Wongee, my beautiful grandma

I came to your widow's heart
Nine months after he was gone
Your grief still raw and open
My infancy your hope
Your arms my cradle
Your round mahogany mirror
Using your hairbrush as a microphone
Late-night fairy tales
I was always the pig with the brick house
Protected from the big bad wolf
Summer ice cream cones and Sunday donuts
Homemade flour noodles
Chicken broth boiling in your thick iron pot
Your call "Woo, hoo, hoo, hoo" every time I came to your front door
Hours in the backyard swing
Climbing your old eucalyptus tree
Carving hearts in its smooth scented bark
Mud pies with candles
You don't remember much now
Your clear blue eyes blind
I'll love you forever
I see your end and wish we could erase time

BUGS AND WINDSHIELDS
About my late brother Justin Jon

Your cheerful hello, your hearty, deep laugh
I quieted the dogs in the background
Snacked on chocolate
Balanced the phone on my shoulder
I complained, you listened
We made plans to see each other
Four days just for us
I marked the calendar
Then you changed the plan
Left ahead of me to heaven
I wasn't ready to lose you
The last thing you said
"Heidi, just face it, sometimes you're the bug
Sometimes you're the windshield"

Life should have given you more windshields

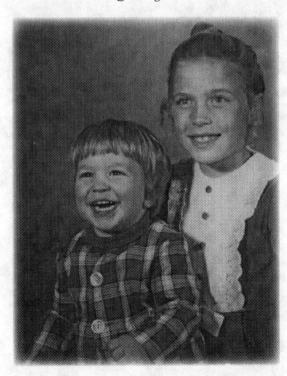

PRISONERS OF WAR

We did not ask to be drafted
Too young to enter this foreign landscape
How much more blood will spill?
Prisoners of a microscopic war
We face the same enemy
We have learned
To sidestep the land mines
Pull our wounded to higher ground
Heal the broken
Try the newest plan of attack
We flash forward
And back
We mourn amputations and bury our dead
Dig our trenches
Hold our breath
Never wanting to surrender

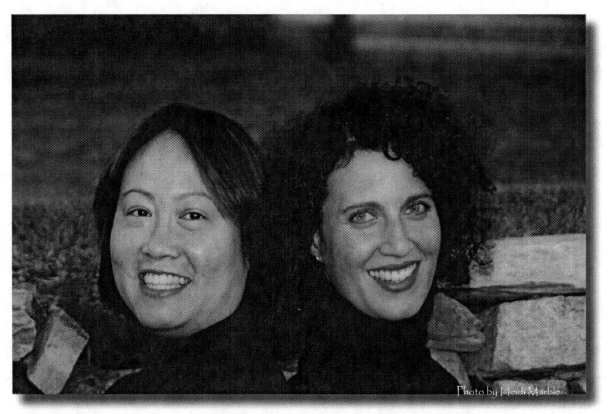

Photo by Heidi Marble

Kimberly Lee Adamson

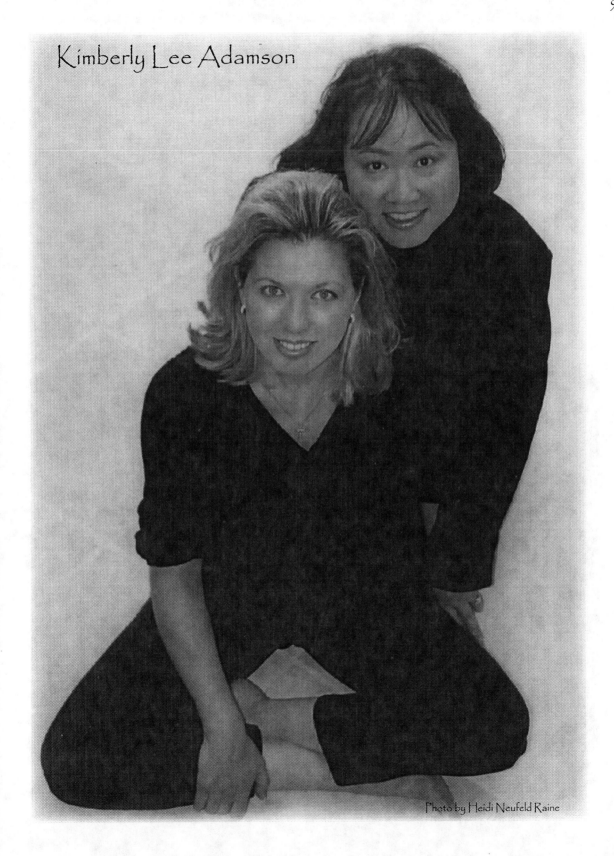

Photo by Heidi Neufeld Raine

ANGELS NEAR
Dedicated to Kathleen, Susan and Rachel

They dragged my wounded body to their souls
Fed me from their flowered china plates
Came into my room
Sat by my side, never showing their fear
I knew they were holy
That kind of love can only be divine
When I was shivering
They wrapped me in their warm downy wings
As I faded
They called me back
With knocks on the door, the ringing phone
They whispered, "You can, you will live."

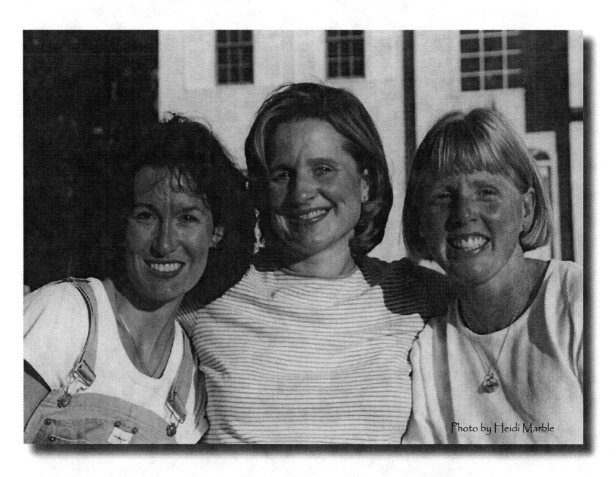

Photo by Heidi Marble

Part Seven

Reflections

When I was tossed like a stone into the ocean of a terminal diagnosis, I sunk to the cold, dark abyss of despair. My only thoughts were of resurfacing and finding a way to reach the shore of hope. I couldn't see the ripples of pain that extended out to my family and friends, the ones who helped pull me in. I asked some of them to write a reflection for my book. As I have read their reflections, I have been able to see the effect that my cancer has had on them. At the same time, each reflection has poured over me like a wave, washing away my pain. I pray that they did the same for my family and friends as they wrote them.

I believe that my husband's contribution, "I Remember," is the most poignant page in this book. When I read it, I sunk into grief. His words gave us the chance to face the pain we had submerged for so long. He, unlike any other person, weathered this storm with quiet strength. He held me in his arms when I could no longer stay afloat. He refused to believe that I would die.

I REMEMBER
By Troy Marble

I remember my wife's voice crying on the doctor's phone
I remember the drive
I remember not knowing what cancer was
I remember hugging a doctor and weeping
I remember his hope for five years
I remember holding her that night
I remember holding my son that night
I remember calling my parents and breaking down
I remember the tests and the waiting
I remember asking why
I remember the poison
I remember the vomiting
I remember her hair in the drain
I remember the baldness
I remember the doctor telling us our son would not have a sister or brother
I remember the long drive to work, crying both ways
I remember being afraid and angry
I remember the biopsies and the blood
I remember the surgery and seeing for the first time
I remember the scars and the drains
I remember the loneliness
I remember the help from friends and family
I remember the helplessness of watching
I remember the burns and the blisters
I remember the pain and the fear
I remember the drugs and the side effects
I remember passing five years
I remember getting trust and hope back
I remember how we were
I remember how lucky I am to still have her
I remember it every day
I will always remember

REFLECTION
By Joy Hamilton, my mom

When I received my precious Heidi's fatal phone call telling me that she was diagnosed with breast cancer, I went through absolute denial. I was sure that it wasn't true--not my child. My child was vital, healthy and filled with love. It could not be my daughter. My daughter was perfect in mind and body, perfect in every way.

My second thought was to rush back to Boston, hold her in my arms and kiss her, making all the bad go away. After all, it always worked when she was little. Slowly, as my mind accepted that this diagnosis was real, that it was correct, I knew beyond a doubt that she would beat the disease.

I did go to Boston to help support my daughter emotionally and to care for my two-year-old grandson and son-in-law. My days there were busy doing laundry, cooking and helping out with other practical tasks. I tried to be a silent strength of support, but nightly I would wake up from a sound sleep, sobbing. The grief, fear and anger were always just below the surface. I rarely cried in front of Heidi; at the time I felt that the best help I could be was to be an example of strength for her--and strong she was.

The greatest terror we have as parents is of something that threatens our children. It attacks the center of our very being, and we feel what they feel--the desperation, pain and fear. Truly, Heidi is half my soul, my being, my reason to survive, my life's sparkle.

All the prayers for Heidi from so many people have helped to bring back the vibrant, loving human being she has always been. She's truly an inspiration as a friend, wife, mother and daughter. How blessed we all are to have witnessed this journey of a miracle in the making and to have been a part of this story of human will, strength, courage and the love of friends and family. How proud I am to call such a wonder my precious daughter.

REFLECTION
By Heidi Neufeld Raine
Photographer and friend

I got to know Heidi in the late 1990s when our husbands were both transferred to Boston to build a bridge over the Charles River. We had each just had baby boys (my third, her first), and we used to joke that our husbands should have married each other because of the long work hours and their obsessive need to debrief with the other via their cell phones every day on their respective commutes home. Little did we know what kind of turn that debriefing would eventually take.

It was during one of those phone calls that we learned Heidi had cancer. She was the first young person to whom I was remotely close to be diagnosed with cancer, and she was given the worst possible diagnosis. I thought it was a death sentence.

I was taking a photography course at the time, and although I don't remember whose idea it was to document her treatment through photos, we were both enthusiastic from the start. She told me later that she had wanted to leave the pictures as a legacy to her son.

Now the pictures serve a different purpose. Maybe they prove what was real, because to meet Heidi today, you might not believe what she went through. It is no longer unbelievable to me that she has recovered--it is harder to believe she was sick. The year she went through treatment has faded into fog, interrupted by only a few clear memories: how very shrunken she was after surgery, the sight of that ghastly box they put in her chest to deliver the medicine, the brokenhearted cries of her son when I buckled him into my car to try to give Heidi a break (he never wanted to leave her). We have the pictures to prove that it happened. But even pictures are deceptive. When I look back and see how thin she was at times, how pale, I think, But I don't remember her that way.

Heidi directed the photos. Whereas I might have tried to put together a stark and somber collection showing a bald and bare-faced woman, she wanted to put on party dresses; she wanted to build nests; she wanted butterflies and costumes. Even my photography instructor said, "See if she'll take off her makeup." But that's not the cancer patient Heidi wanted to be. For the sake of a photo, she climbed trees; she lay naked on cold floors; she tied pill bottles to her fingers, laughing all the while. If you hear her entire story, you will realize that nothing in Heidi's life has ever happened without drama. She may think cancer has changed her, but just recently, I came home to a message from her on my answering machine: "Heidi, it's Heidi. I had an idea for the front cover. I thought we could build a cocoon."

Heidi, you haven't changed. You are, you were and you always will be exuberance itself, and I love you. Keep these pictures to remind you, but know that they, like the jewels on your mannequins, are best seen as part of something more. It is in putting all your pieces together, the brassy with the gold, the shiny with the matte, that we can see you whole.

REFLECTION
By Mary Pat Reeves

When I met my dear friend Heidi in 1991, I was intimidated by her beauty. But although she always looked gorgeous on the outside, her insides were constantly giving her grief. I've affectionately referred to her as a lemon--she looks great, but she doesn't run very well.

I visited Heidi six months before her diagnosis, and she knew something else was wrong. Something different. When I heard it was cancer, I just couldn't believe she'd been dealt yet another rotten hand, this one being the worst. I felt so helpless. I wanted so much to be with her, but I had a newborn and a toddler, and a trip from Phoenix to Boston at that time would have been nearly impossible. It did my heart good to know that her selfless neighbors, family, and friends in the area were doing everything they could to help.

Since that fateful diagnosis day in April of 2000, Heidi's birthday has become very precious to me. Her fortieth was one I'll never forget. I can only imagine what my beautiful friend has had to endure over the last six years, but I do know that she is the most plucky, courageous, stubborn, feisty, eloquent woman I know. I've been so amazed and inspired by how she has dealt with her illness. I know that her book will be a godsend to those feeling the isolation and loneliness of dealing with breast cancer. I feel incredibly blessed to be able to call Heidi Marble my friend.

REFLECTION
By Cordetta Spells
Photographer

Anyone who knows me well knows that it is rare for me to ever have difficulty finding words to say (whether they are the best choice to use at that moment or not). Heidi has managed to do just that for me! How many ways can you describe beauty, truth, love and honor? All of these make up her mind, body and spirit. She is the first person I've ever met who has truly managed to create beauty out of the ugliest and saddest conditions through her gifts as a teacher, poet and mannequin jewelry artist.

Anyone who knows me well also knows that when I do manage to "find the words," I have no problem telling it as I see it. First of all, I have come to know Heidi pretty well over these past few months, and I can truly say I love her very much. Maybe because I see so much of myself in her at times (the truly nice part of myself, that is). But there was also a part of her that concerned me—her determination and drive to get this great work accomplished, which is great until it becomes a destination driven by fear. In her zest and appreciation for the life that was given back to her, Heidi became driven by the true fear that she would not be around to see it all come to fruition (something that none of us has any control over).

As Heidi and I talked about her fear one day, we both agreed that God would not have brought her this far in life without letting her realize her dream to help others live and fulfill theirs. She then told me that there was something I'd mentioned in a recent news article that made her feel less anxious and more enlightened about life and death. An inspirational gift for her, so I will share it with you.

It the news article about an upcoming benefit for hospice, I mentioned that it was easy for me to believe that there was no reason to be concerned about death's transition, as I believe there is an afterlife for me as God has promised. For me, it only makes sense! We were conceived and born from the womb, a water world—a life that we knew of and grew in for only as long as we needed to be. When our time was up and our mission completed, we transitioned into another world, where we live now, unable to return to that other world and having no remembrance of it. So the same shall occur. We will be alive on this earth until we've learned and done what we have been given time to learn and do. When our time here is complete, our purpose fulfilled, once again we will transition to a new and beautiful life.

Heidi, like the name of her company, is UNDONE. She has since "chilled" and, thankfully, realizes that her mission here is not complete. The life she has been given continues to be a blessing for all who meet and share her time.

The idea of Buttons-n-Dollars just came to me as a way to bring attention to Heidi's art (the girlz, as I call them). They were therapy for her through the most trying time of her life. She transformed the blank, thin, lifeless surfaces of her mannequins into works of art--a metamorphosis not unlike that of a butterfly, not unlike that of herself. In all, no two pieces of Heidi's art are alike; they are all beautiful and something to behold. I thought Heidi should start a campaign where people can send buttons and jewelry attached to dollars. In turn she could use the trinkets to create new girlz and the dollars to help cancer patients. The new girlz could eventually be displayed, sold and auctioned off, in turn generating even more for Buttons-N-Dollars. The possibilities for expansion are endless.

Heidi continues to amaze me and honor me. It started with a visit to her classroom, where my daughter was her student. She had seen my photo business card and portfolio, and after her fountain of tears dried up from being touched by my work, she asked if I'd shoot her family's portrait. (I was really flattered that she cried, until I found out that she cries when a leaf falls off a tree. So much for the ol' ego!)

These past months our friendship and photographic duties have grown. Now she has honored me not only by including me in her life and project but also by asking me to write something she thinks people would care to read. I guess if you gotten this far, she was right, and I thank you.

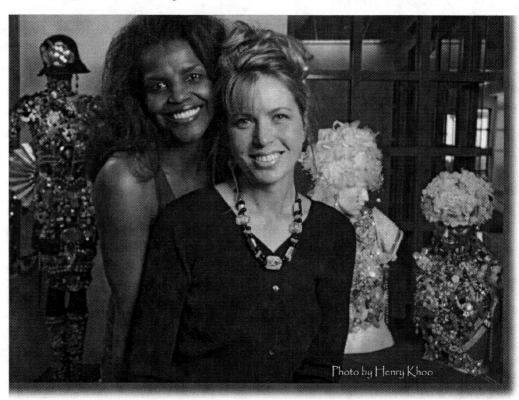

Photo by Henry Khoo

SYNCHRONICITY
By Kathie Kalafatis
Fellow philanthropist and friend

Heidi's and my journey together began when our sons were in the same kindergarten class in the fall of 2003. I couldn't have known that bright, sunny day in September that our meeting would bring such purpose into my life. When I met Heidi, I discovered a reflection of my soul in her. I believe that people attract certain people to their lives without effort and in perfect synchronicity. Like creating a grid of our life experiences in the physical and the realization that we share common paths with others. When Heidi first told me that she was a breast cancer survivor, it shocked me, for she exuded such a healthy glow and vitality around her.

When traveling along life's path, we sometimes forget that we are not alone. Heidi and I have found that we share many common experiences. In the first years of my son's life, when the world was changing around me and I had to face my own health fears, it never occurred to me that another first-time mom was facing hers. For Heidi, this was the battle of her life against an unforgiving disease--breast cancer. The day I baptized my daughter and released butterflies into the air as a symbol of rebirth, it never occurred to me how important butterflies were to someone I was yet to know. Heidi has survived the battle against a deadly enemy and has emerged from her own cocoon.

In 2006, we celebrated New Year's together. Like many people, we talked about our wishes and desires for the new year. We wanted to do something outside of ourselves to help others. It was at that time that Heidi mentioned to me that she wanted to start up a charity foundation named Buttons-n-Dollars to benefit breast cancer patients who could not afford to continue with their treatments. Breast cancer had always been a silent fear I struggled with since my own grandmother had a mastectomy at age forty-four. From the moment Heidi told me this, I knew I wanted to help her, and like two birds synchronized in flight, we took off into the world of philanthropy.

During our first discussions, we came up with an idea for a fashion show benefiting breast cancer patients. This would allow Heidi to showcase her mannequins in a diva setting and allow breast cancer patients and survivors to strut their stuff down the catwalk. A couple of weeks into our planning, a newly found friend, Kathy, called to invite me to a charity event she was attending. I was really surprised to hear it was a fashion show and it was being held in our local community. I immediately asked if I could invite my good friend Heidi, as we were in the midst of planning our own fashion-show charity event. Of course she said yes and was excited about helping introduce us to people who would be beneficial to our cause. We attended the event, and more things continued to fall into place.

During the event, Heidi and I toured the room, looking at purses that were on display for auction. We both spotted a beautiful, black, beaded purse with butterfly embroidery. Our eyes lit up with anticipation as we dropped our tickets into the box and waited for the announcement. When it appeared that all of the purses had been handed out and we were getting ready to leave for home, a woman approached us from across the room and asked if either of us was Kathie. I had in fact won the purse! I decided to give the purse to Heidi as a gift symbolizing our friendship. It seemed so fitting for her to have it. After all, the butterfly has long been known as a symbol of physical existence. Butterflies are strong enough to endure the metamorphosis of change, yet so fragile that they can be torn apart by an intense rain. Heidi thought it would be a good idea to use the purse as a "traveling purse"; we would leave special notes inside it for one another, telling of our great purse adventures.

Winning the purse was no mistake. It is another evidence of synchronicity between us, hiding in the shadows of our souls that are interconnected with a tiny thread spread over many years. Our common threads were woven together long before our paths crossed, leading up to the inevitable union of two souls evolving together for a purpose much greater than ourselves. Synchronicity is something that happens against all odds, something that the Universe seems to move into place to fill our inner needs.

Through Heidi's experiences, I've become more aware of my own exalted level of consciousness, which has helped me develop my intuition about myself and others. Heidi has shown me that in a world full of propaganda that perpetuates the idea that our body image equates with our self-image, we are not the sum of our body parts, but of our human nature. It is Heidi's beautiful spirit that touches everyone she meets. It is her courage and strength that we all draw from, and it is her devotion to helping others that truly inspires us. I can't help but be thankful that meeting Heidi was part of my life's path and believe that we were fated to be friends.

REFLECTION
By Kathleen Rocco

Heidi and I met as backyard neighbors in a small town in Massachusetts. We became close friends; she was like the sister I never had growing up. We shared everything—dinner and vacations, laughter and advice. Even our sons were the best of friends!

Cancer, breast cancer, was something I had thought would never touch my life or the life of someone so near and dear to me. It had once before, so never did I think it would happen again. So when, during a typical, lazy afternoon outside watching our children play, Heidi said that something was not right with her breast and that she was going to see a specialist, denial, ignorance and optimism caused me to say quickly, "It will be fine, Heidi." In fact, it turned out to be anything but fine.

Tears still fill my eyes as I recall Heidi and Troy sitting with me and telling me about Heidi's diagnosis of inflammatory breast cancer and her chances of survival. Inside I crumbled as they described the days that lay ahead for them and Heidi asked me if I would help her husband care for their child, Blake. In shock, I struggled to find words to console. I couldn't understand and believe how someone so young, so vibrant and so healthy could be suffering from such a horrible disease. It wasn't comprehendible, nor was it fair.

Heidi's group of close friends worked hard to be strong for Heidi and her family, who were strong themselves. We all had a different strength and role we used to care for them. One of us understood and interpreted the medical information; another endlessly empathized and brought comfort with words and relaxing meditation; and yet another provided for the basic needs of the family, such as meals and child care. All the while we supported each other. Helping Heidi and her family in our own ways helped us to get through this difficult time by being actively involved.

Caring for Heidi became the focus of every day, but it still did not take away the overwhelming sadness, anger, helplessness and lack of control that I felt. I remember waking every night and every morning for a very long time, hoping I had just had a very bad dream. It saddened me deeply that Heidi had to suffer so terribly physically and that she had to face the likelihood that she would not see her cherished son become an adult. This same sadness struck me as I thought about Heidi's husband and son watching her pain and sadness. My emotions vacillated between sadness and anger and would bring me to tears so often. It made me feel a vulnerability I had never experienced before.

Cancer brought immeasurable pain and suffering to Heidi and her family and friends. But we have all been given a gift of learning to appreciate life more. It has been six years since Heidi's diagnosis, and Heidi's beautiful blonde hair and her vibrancy, glimmer and smile are back to stay. Our bond is stronger than ever before, and Heidi continues to make an invaluable difference in the lives of so many!

REFLECTION
By Roger Marble

When I first heard about Heidi's illness, I was driving down the freeway speaking with Troy, my brother. I've never really watched a grown man cry, but listening to one from 3,000 miles away broke my heart. Troy is my best friend in the world, and hearing the sound in his voice made this far too real. My first reaction was not just to wonder about Heidi, but also to be concerned about what would happen to Troy and Blake. Obviously, Troy could not care for his new son and work at the same time.

I am so grateful that Heidi is a little bit of a worrier (no offense meant); however, without her persistence, this disease may never have been diagnosed. Heidi actually refused to take no for an answer. After I read so many web sites that address inflammatory breast cancer, it was apparent that the number one cause of death was ignoring the rash or discoloration that typically comes with this disease. It is simply amazing how many women who I've spoken to about this have never heard of inflammatory breast cancer or the signs that help to diagnose it. I hope that Heidi's story will help other women to recognize symptoms of this dreadful disease and allow them and their families a second chance at life.

I, along with my family and friends, are so honored to have Heidi back in our lives and healthy again. We love you, Heidi, Troy and Blake.

REFLECTION
By Denise Baker Fisher, CRNA
David P. Fisher, MD

Heidi and I met because of an ad for a house rental in 2001; it was a divine appointment. Heidi had recently finished her treatment, entering into that abyss of waiting--waiting, wondering and hoping that this monster called cancer won't return. She, like so many of us who have had cancer, was trying to embrace life again, yet was dragging a ten-pound weight of fear behind her. I had been in that place after I was diagnosed with treatable breast cancer eight years before, and I had made friends with it in many ways. We were able to share our fears and thoughts as we fought our common enemy. We eventually entered a three-day breast cancer walk together, which was an encouraging time for both of us as we marched with so many sisters in the fight.

Recently I discovered that my cancer had metastasized; it was the first time in my life that I could not personally fix my own problem. As a nurse anesthetist married to a general surgeon, I understood the limitations of Western medicine in treating my disease. I was offered chemotherapy with the hopes that it would prolong my life and buy me some time, but my husband and I decided to walk away from all Western medicine had to offer. We made a choice to believe the Word of God, the Bible. In it, God is called Jehovah-Rapha, the God who heals. I began to read and meditate daily on the healings of Jesus. This strengthened my faith to believe that God, who says that He is the same yesterday, today and forever (Hebrews 13:8), would heal me as He healed then. God also directed me to go to a holistic nutritionist to help me detoxify my body. I am doing my part in this battle by supplying my body with healthy, organic foods, nutrient-rich vegetable juices, clean water and rest.

I have had vast improvement during this past year. The tumors are dramatically reduced in size, and I had complete resolution of a pulmonary effusion. I am confident that I will see complete healing of this disease in my body.

The message I bring is one of HOPE. No verdict by an oncologist is final. There are many paths to healing, but all healing comes from God. He can heal in a second or He can use holistic medicine, with or without Western medicine. Each of us must take responsibility for our paths to wellness and battle against cancer in ways that resonate in our souls. A large community of people who have found healing after a terminal diagnosis exists. We can learn so much from them. Let's trust God and trust how He is leading us. Let's believe that we can be healed!

REFLECTION
By Susan Bauer-Wu, DNSc, RN Dana-Farber Cancer Institute

What a privilege it was for me to walk with Heidi when cancer first shook up her life. Nearly every month we spent two hours together at a lovely oasis for cancer patients called Hope Lodge, where I co-led a support group, Path to Healing with Cancer, with my colleague and friend Elana Rosenbaum. This was clearly one of those circumstances when it's not the quantity of time, but the quality, that makes the difference. Every time we met at Hope Lodge progress was made.

Seeds of transformation were planted in rich, fertile soil-Heidi arrived at our group with a sincere commitment and receptivity to nurture her spirit and to learn and grow. Quieting the mind through mindful meditation, stretching the body through gentle yoga and creatively expressing herself through art and writing—these were the water and fertilizer to nourish the growing seed. Most important were genuine presence, authentic caring and sharing, tears of sadness and love and laughter—they provided light and warmth to catalyze growth. I witnessed a fragile, scared seedling gradually blossom into a vibrant, beautiful flower with deep roots, a strong stem and bright colors all her own. Heidi's personal transformation over that two-year period was simply magnificent.

As I look back at this special time with Heidi, I vividly recall the angst she experienced: profound, heartfelt sadness, anger and fear. Even more indelible on my mind was how she acknowledged and expressed her emotional and physical pain. Rather than pushing it away, she allowed herself to feel whatever she felt and to let these feelings flow through spoken and written words, drawing and clay molding, moving her body and playing the piano.

I will never forget Heidi's last group meeting with us before she moved away to the West Coast. She sat at the piano and played a song that she had composed. We listened in awe, our skin tingled, and tears of love gently flowed from our eyes. The music was extraordinarily beautiful. We were taken aback to find out that Heidi learned to play the piano only after her diagnosis with breast cancer. Somehow, having cancer allowed her to tap into a hidden talent: A new self-confidence and new ways of expressing herself were born.

REFLECTION
By Kimberly Lee Adamson

As I walk into my first cancer support group, I am struck by how we all look alike. Despite being of different ages and ethnicities, cancer has made us all look sterilely similar. Because of the absence of our facial hair and the smoothness of our skin, not even a blemish surviving the pool of toxins we call chemotherapy, we look like mannequins! We are anonymous, stripped of our identities. However, as the group begins, I am struck by the beauty and radiant life that shines forth from one particular "cancer patient." As she speaks, I hear humor; I hear fear; I hear relief. Most of all, I hear honesty--raw, uncensored and felt to the core. She has finished her first round of chemotherapy and has just had bilateral mastectomies. The similarities in our stories make me want to know her more.

So began my life with Heidi, and from that day on, my life has been blessed by her friendship. As time went by, we continued to learn about each other through our support group and over the phone. In our support group, Heidi read her poetry, which always poignantly put to words the raw emotions of this devastating illness. She wrote of loss, anger, joy, despair and hope. Her words shook the fortress of my defenses. Her courage in trying to make sense of cancer and all that had happened to her encouraged me to enter that scary space of my interior life. In our darkest hours, our souls could meet as kindred spirits. Her humor incarnate in Matilda, our fearless leader and icon, balanced the darker hours and brought hope to our bonded friendship. Over the phone we continued to share laughter, tears, anger, fear, the unknown and hope. Both of us have been robbed of so much in our marriage, sexuality and life.

Despite the physical distance, our friendship has continued. I recall the last time we met together before Heidi left the East Coast. We revealed our scars to each other. Other than my husband and my health care team, I had not shown my scars to anyone. I remember the comparisons, the respect, the sadness and the sacredness. We had entered a friendship forged by scars.

Though now we live on opposite coasts, our friendship continues to transcend all other friendships. It's as if seeing and living in our nakedness have bonded us for life. Though we now look different from how we looked the first day we met, we are still bonded in friendship by the scars that lie beneath the visible changes.

You see, while I reflect on my experience of Heidi's cancer, I can't help but recall all that makes Heidi a special person. She is not the cancer. She is not all that has happened to her because of cancer. Heidi, like a phoenix rising above the ashes of her despair, has become for me a symbol of hope, of all things beautiful and of life after death. To me she is pure Love.

REFLECTION
By Yasemine Turkman

I remember when we first met. It was in the spring of 2000 in Hester Hill's support group for women who had been newly diagnosed with breast cancer at the Beth Israel Deaconess Medical Center. You were wearing a funky overalls outfit and on your head were a bandana and a straw hat. It was hard to believe you were going through chemotherapy at the time and had no hair—to me, you radiated such beauty that your face shone (or perhaps that was a hot flash!).

Over the next few months, we became close friends. Kimberly joined the support group and the three of us just seemed to stick together. We were young for the group. Most of the other women were postmenopausal, but there we were, in our early 30s with so much life yet to live. Even though we shared youth, we were at very different stages in our lives. You were married with a young child. Kimberly was engaged and had postponed the wedding due to treatment. I was single. We also had different cancer histories and different types of breast cancer. Despite our dissimilarities and our recent acquaintanceship, you and Kimberly very quickly became my greatest sources of support.

Many of my healthy friends seemed to have a difficult time understanding the cancer experience. Some even withdrew. I never expected to have received the strength I did from you and Kimberly, given that we were each fighting for our lives. Yet somehow we clung together. I have this image of the three of us—people severely compromised yet leaning on each other to function as a whole.

One of the fun times I remember is going to Hope Lodge for the monthly program, Path to Healing with Cancer. We would meet early for dinner, and the laughter would start. Then at Hope Lodge, our giggles would just intensify. We were talking about some pretty serious stuff, such as death and pain, but somehow doing it together made it all the more bearable. The connection buoyed me, and I always left feeling light.

I'll never forget the road trip we took to Maine. When a follow-up mammogram had revealed a new spot on my breast, I wanted a second opinion from Dr. Dixie Mills at the Women to Women Clinic in Yarmouth. We drove up a day early and spent the evening with your friends Julie and Dan in their charming log home. We had the luxury of a dip in the hot tub under a starlit, New England, March sky. What a relief it was to learn that the spot was benign! Your presence comforted me during a very trying time.

At this point, I must mention our dear friend Matilda. It was on our way to

Maine that you introduced me to this pink, plastic-flamingo lawn ornament that would come to represent the true bonds of friendship. Whenever you, Kimberly or I was going through a difficult time, Matilda would show up to bring smiles to our faces and to remind us that we were not alone.

Then there was the retreat at Innisfree. What a beautiful weekend in the nature of New Hampshire! Kimberly couldn't make it, so Matilda came along in her place. I also remember the interesting sounds that came from our neighbor's room—some morning ritual that involved howling. Whatever it was, it was contagious, because we ended up howling in laughter and diving into our pillows to stifle the noise!

I was heartbroken when you moved to California. While I was happy for the opportunities that awaited you and your family, I knew I would miss you terribly. It was such a joy to come and visit you. It felt like no time had passed and our connection was just as strong as before. We danced to the Bee Gees' "Staying Alive" as we had the night of Kimberly's wedding. Kimberly wasn't there, but we called her and danced with the phone!

Well, my dear friend, thank you for the precious gift of your friendship. I know that no matter how far we may be or how long it has been since we have spoken, the connection runs deep. I carry you close to my heart always!

I am just thrilled with your creativity and wish you much joy, health and prosperity!

REFLECTION
By Julie McQueen

I first met Heidi at a 1997 New Year's Eve gathering at my home in Massachusetts. We seemed to hit it off immediately. Her husband and mine were working together on the bridge project that brought Heidi and her family to Boston, and I worked for the same company.

A few weeks before we met, my mom (Marilyn, whom Heidi has graciously acknowledged) was diagnosed with breast cancer for the second time, after three and one-half years in remission. Little did Heidi and I know that cancer would eventually be a common thread in our lives.

My mom was preparing to receive stem cell treatment when it was discovered that the breast cancer had spread to her brain. We wanted to be able to spend as much time with her as possible, and we were granted the ability to do so. In August 1998 my husband and I quit the company that had been such a big part of our lives for so long fifteen and seventeen years respectively). My mom spent some time with us in Massachusetts during her last couple of years, and it always included visits with Heidi and her family. Heidi and my mom developed a truly special bond during that time. Needless to say, it was a shock when Heidi was diagnosed with breast cancer in April 2000. Though my mom's condition had worsened, my mom would pray for Heidi and her family, and would assure me that it would all be okay. Though Heidi had started her own arduous journey, Heidi continued to support me and to be a true friend. My relationships with my mom and Heidi included plenty of laughter and smiles, in spite of whatever else was taking place.

My mom died on September 11, 2000. My husband and I had spent a good part of the last six weeks of her life in Wisconsin, helping to care for her. Just hours before my mom died, Heidi called me, as if she knew exactly what I needed and when, to "check in" and to let us know that she was thinking of us. I called her back with the news a few hours later, grateful for the connection.

In spite of the fearful situation that each woman faced, neither ever shrank from supporting their family and friends. They both exemplified selfless courage I will always remember how Heidi helped me when I returned home, exhausted, during the last phase of my mother's illness. In spite of what she was dealing with herself, Heidi had prepared and delivered an entire meal, which was waiting for us in our refrigerator. She is living proof that God always provides what we need, even if it is not quite the way we envision it. Frequently it is much better! I am honored to be Heidi's friend and am grateful to be given an opportunity to reflect on such a memorable time of my life with such fondness.

REFLECTION
By Elana Rosenbaum, MS, LICSW
Author of *Here For Now*

To have cancer is to be challenged in mind and body. It can be devastating or it can be an opportunity to reach new realms of emotional honesty and strength. When I met Heidi for the first time at Hope Lodge, where a group of people touched by cancer came together and meditated, laughed, cried, drew pictures and told stories, I remember being struck by Heidi's beauty and radiance of spirit. She was bald and her body was scarred, but her eyes shone and she always wore beautiful colorful, clothes that reflected her inner courage and daring. Heidi faced what arose inside of her and named it but moved with it in a way that helped us all join together and transcend fear and self-pity. Her aliveness lit the group and sparked us to deeper expressions of love and hope even in the midst of despair.

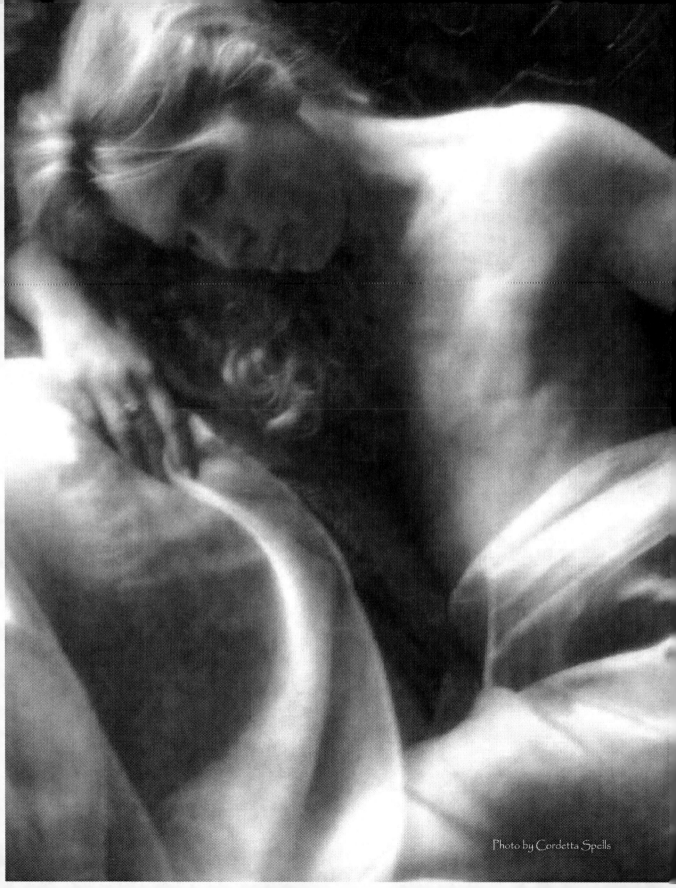

Photo by Cordetta Spells

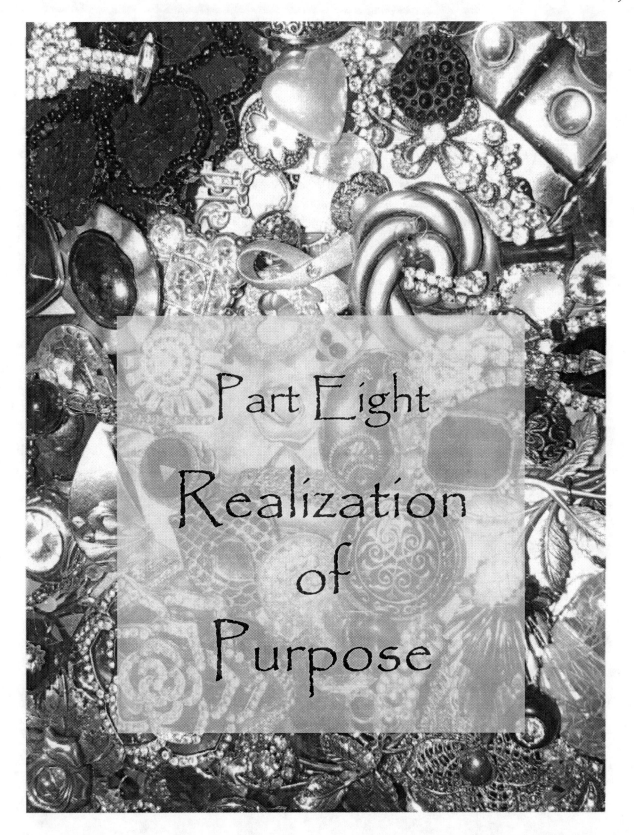

Part Eight

Realization of Purpose

The last part of this book truly captures the purpose I have harnessed. This section begins with *Thunder* written by Ezio Lucido. The first night we interviewed, I told him about the "calling" I had experienced. He then explained his theory on purpose and how it manifests in a human being. I asked him to write down every word so I would never forget. I hope his reflections on lightning and thunder touch your heart as much they have touched mine.

We reworked the end of the book at the last minute because I received a beautiful gift. Cordetta presented me with an album of all the pictures she has taken over the last few months. I was brought to tears by these images and understood that her photographs will tell the story my words never could. The final pages are filled with the birth of my purpose.

How did I arrive at this revelation? My fortieth birthday came and went with celebration, but I still felt I didn't fully comprehend what I was supposed to do with the person I had evolved into. Cancer was a harsh teacher with many painful lessons. It didn't seem like enough to pretend the experience didn't change me.

During my treatment, someone gave me a bracelet made out of old buttons. I was fascinated by this tiny creation and the resourcefulness behind it. It made me consider how many ways we can use our lives that aren't obvious. I wanted to recreate these bracelets for my friends. I quickly learned that sewing and needles were not my cup of tea. Instead I started to create picture frames, mirrors, hats and boxes using a glue gun. I expanded my buttons to broken bits and pieces of old jewelry, watches, pins and belt buckles that I would find at junk stores. Soon people were giving me their unused trinkets. With every item I made and make a watch and angel are included. The watch is for more time and the angel is for blessings.

Several years passed and we moved to California and I was still enamored with this hobby. Then one day while I was scavenger hunting, I saw a bald, damaged mannequin that no one wanted. I immediately related to this pathetic form. I purchased the mannequin, carried her out to my car. Then the antics of trying to fit her in my sedan started. I held my head up high as I tried to remove her arms and legs. After what seemed like hours, she finally ended up in the passenger seat. Of course, I didn't have a blanket or anything to cover her up with. I drove home trying not to make eye contact with the people staring at me.

Once I got her home, the staring continued as my son, husband and dogs took in this new creature. Angel was barking and her hair was standing on end. Troy was shaking his head and Blake wanted to know what I was planning to do with this lady. I didn't have any answers at the time. I proceeded to clean her and wrap her in a bolt of black elastic. I set her up and I slowly added jewelry and buttons Over the course of three years I created "Jewels."

On a whim, I took her down to a local art gallery for its annual juried art show. Much to my surprise, Jewels won an award. I had a few other mannequins I had collected, and I started working on them. The gallery asked me to display more. Then one day the lightning struck.

After a bout with depression, I came home fresh from my injection at the cancer center. The house was a mess, the answering machine was blinking, the dogs wanted food, people wanted food and I all I wanted was my bed. I touched the Play button on my answering machine and heard the unfamiliar voice of a female reporter inquiring about my artwork. Every cell in my body vibrated and I understood that change was coming. I then turned to my counter where Cordetta had returned the manuscript of my book along with a letter of encouragement. I read the letter and she explained her vision of my starting a grass-roots fundraising campaign where people would donate money along with any old broken jewelry, buttons odds and ends. I would then use the trinkets on my mannequins and give the money to subsidize cancer patients' needs. She thought the campaign should be called Buttons-n-Dollars.

Within five minutes I was inside my purpose, and fully immersed in joy. All the elements came together and I knew how my art could finally be used in a meaningful way. I immediately called Rick Siefke, oncology social worker at North Bay Hospital and told him about the idea. He put me in touch with Brett Johnson, President of the North Bay Health Care Foundation. Brett met with me after hours the next day and we went into action.

From there, I was asked to participate in the North Bay donor recognition event. I displayed my artwork and spoke to the audience about transformation. I didn't feel the least bit nervous, it just felt right. I spoke from the heart, from a place of intention. The magic continued as Ezio unveiled his documentary featuring my story along with the history of philanthropy that preceded me.

The miracles started to flow in a way I never expected. During the first week of my profound realization I sent part of the book manuscript to a publisher. Much to my surprise he accepted the project. Since that time the universe has provided all the right people at all the right times. Now that I am in alignment, everything is falling into place. Aside from meeting my husband nothing has ever felt so right. I don't feel the need to analyze and question where I am headed. I know that just as my wings the plan will unfold .Through my business "Undone" and my book I hope to impact the lives of people dealing with this disease. The art is becoming the public's work in progress. My vision is to have the mannequins displayed at various places around the country.

In closing, I hope that my book reads like a love story about life. No matter if I live one more minute, or fifty more years, I know I have lived. I will not leave this earth with my dreams inside of me. If I have anything to leave you with it is this. Feel all your emotions, you have them for a reason! Remember you are not alone. When in doubt give even if it's just a smile. Don't let fear keep you from trying. No matter what, remember we all have the capacity to fly here and beyond.

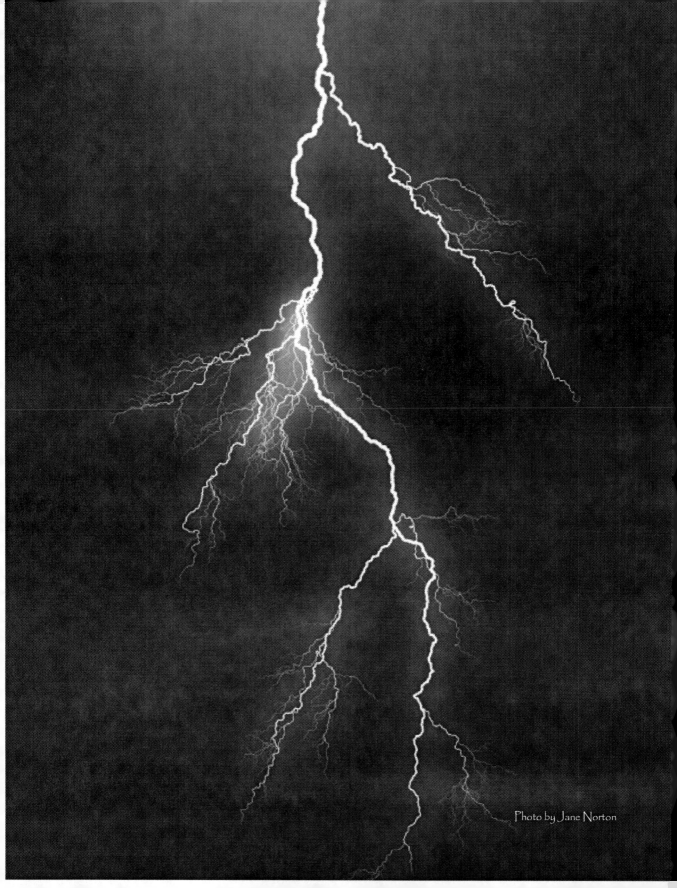

Photo by Jane Norton

THUNDER
By Ezio Lucido, Motion Eclipse Pictures

To me a person's relationship with the universe is much like the relationship between lightning and thunder with the earth. Lightning occurs when air in the clouds rises quickly and then cools, cooling water vapor into raindrops and snowflakes. There is a change in electrical charge when this happens, and thus this charge, or lighting bolt, strikes between the clouds and the ground and sometimes in the air. Lightning causes thunder. When a bolt of lightning travels through air, it increases the temperature to over ten thousand degrees Fahrenheit. This heat causes the air to expand and cool very rapidly, pushing the air out. When the air rushes back into this area around both sides of the lightning bolt, thunder is created. It is the impact of air colliding with air.

So what does all that have to do with the human spirit, and more specifically, what does it have to do with Heidi Marble? I believe that in every human being there are specific, separate elements that make up the whole. For thunder to happen, many things have to occur at the right time in the right place. It is a buildup of specific events. In Heidi, I believe, these elements have come together and today she thunders. It is a mixture of experience, timing, purpose and choice. When the mind, body, heart and soul come together in one place, working together, in synergy, the result is thunder. It is a powerful blend of human potential that ignites into a force that can do good for the world. It is a sound of hope that starts close but travels far.

Cancer crashed into Heidi's life so that she had to look purpose in the face. The cancer was like lightning--it was a charge rushing through her life, heating the vision of herself in this world well over tens of thousands of degrees. She separated herself from herself much like the air does on either side of a lightning strike. Heidi's dimensions--her heart, her mind, her body and her soul--were separated by this strike of lightning, allowing her to see these elements that make up her whole self. Eventually, through the thickening storm clouds, she began to see herself clearer and clearer until, finally, she saw her purpose. At this point, she had to make a choice. Heidi decided to have all of her dimensions return to her center, colliding there and causing thunder.

THUNDER

Pelting drops from angry clouds
The wind slings the dark chime into clanking
Lightning spreads its vascular display across the humid sky
I am not grounded
Standing out in the open
A conduit
Wet and cold
The elements drench me
I smell the damp mesquite branches
Surrounded by power greater than myself
I am struck with purpose
Every cell electrocuted
The dim life I've lived now shines bright
I feel my thunder as the storm rolls away

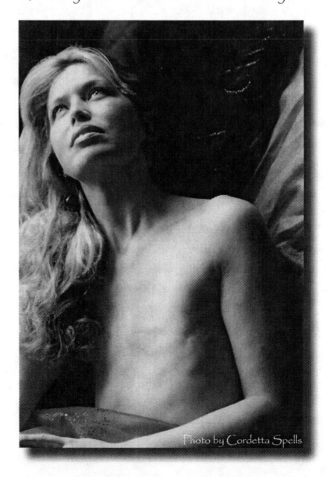

Photo by Cordetta Spells

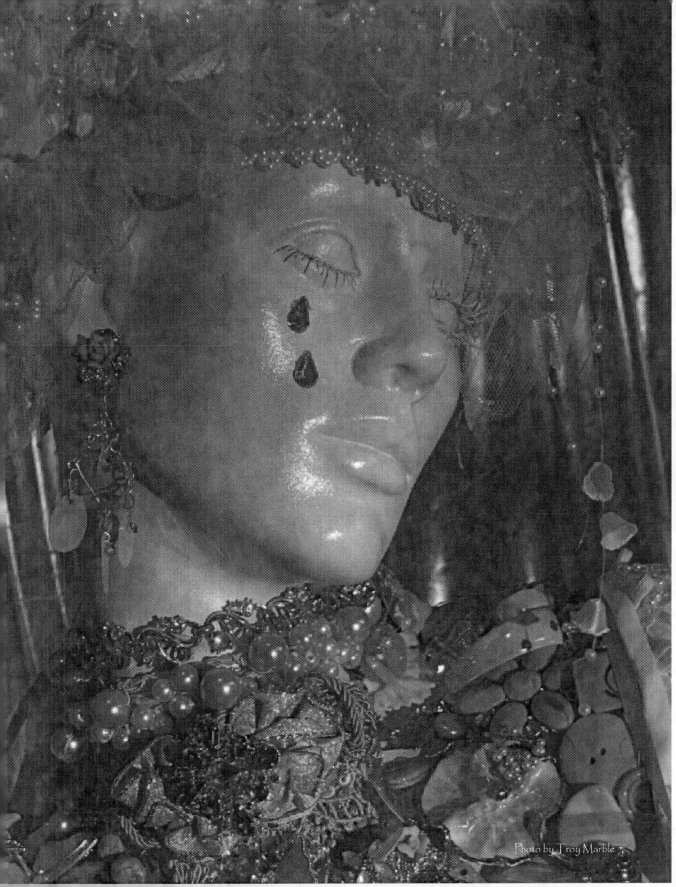

Photo by Troy Marble

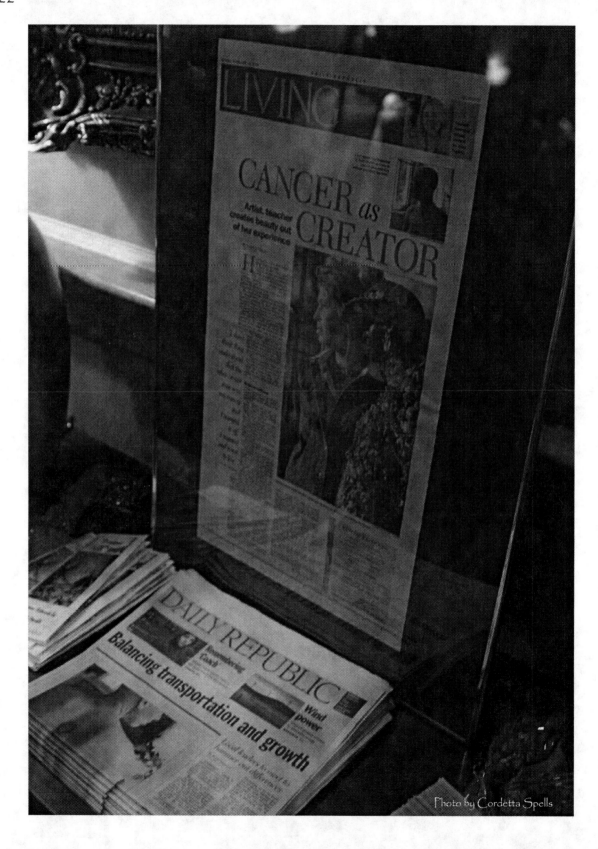

Photo by Cordetta Spells

Buttons-N-Dollars

Creations by Heidi Marble, Cancer Survivor

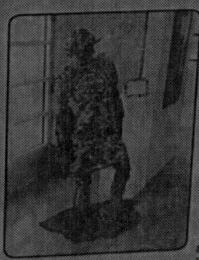

Heidi Marble, a six-year cancer survivor, creates stunning life-size works of art from donated jewelry, buttons, watches and belts. Many of these items may have broken clasps or parts, but that doesn't stop Heidi from creating a new life for them. Often donors include a piece of history with their donation.

"I am honored to share any stories along with my art. Through your donations of old or broken jewelry, buttons, and watches, we can make a difference." Heidi says. Her work is displayed at various locations throughout the Bay Area.

Heidi credits NorthBay Cancer Center and Dr. James Long with a huge part of her healing. Her mission is to bring awareness and funds to the NorthBay Cancer Center. Monetary donations received by *Buttons-N-Dollars* are tax deducible and will be given to the NorthBay Healthcare Foundation for the NorthBay Cancer Center.

Donated funds will be used to subsidize people in our community who cannot afford the treatment they need. "Every day that I am given will be spent pursuing the hope that my fellow travelers will all have the support they deserve," Heidi says.

Donations of jewelry, buttons, watches, and belts should be placed in zip lock bags and given to either a guild volunteer or the front registration desk. For questions, please contact NorthBay Healthcare Foundation at 426-4273.

Please mail any monetary donations to:

Buttons-N-Dollars
750 Pavilion Drive
Fairfield, CA 94534

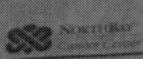

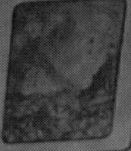

Photo by Cordetta Spells

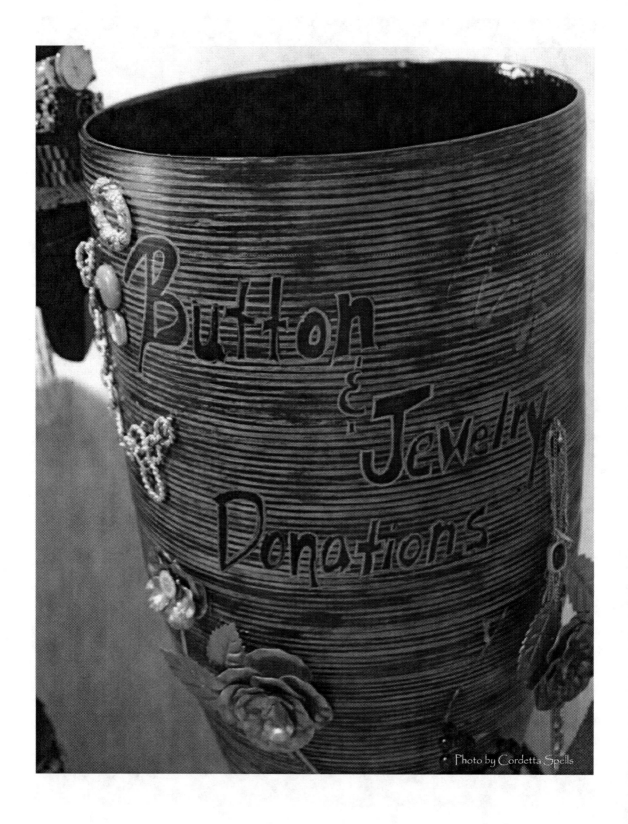

Photo by Cordetta Spells

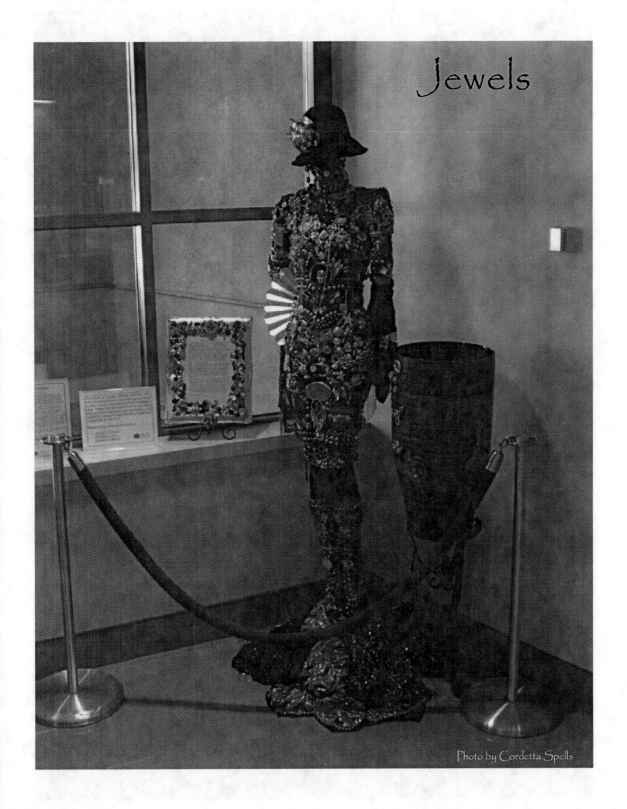

Jewels

Photo by Cordetta Spells

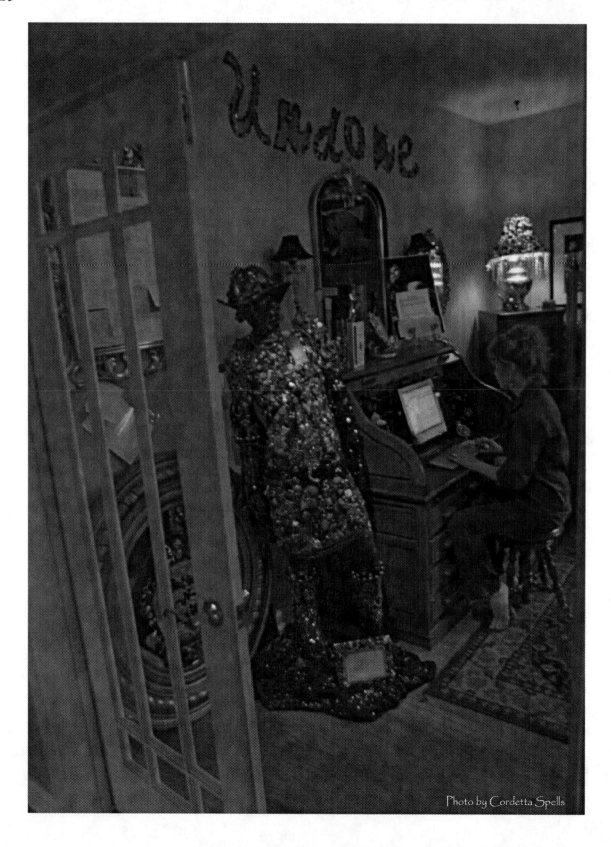

Photo by Cordetta Spells

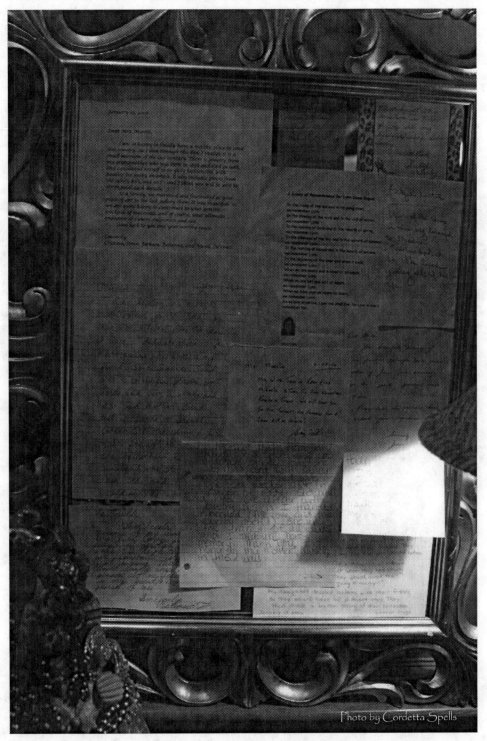

Photo by Cordetta Spells

Letters from Donors

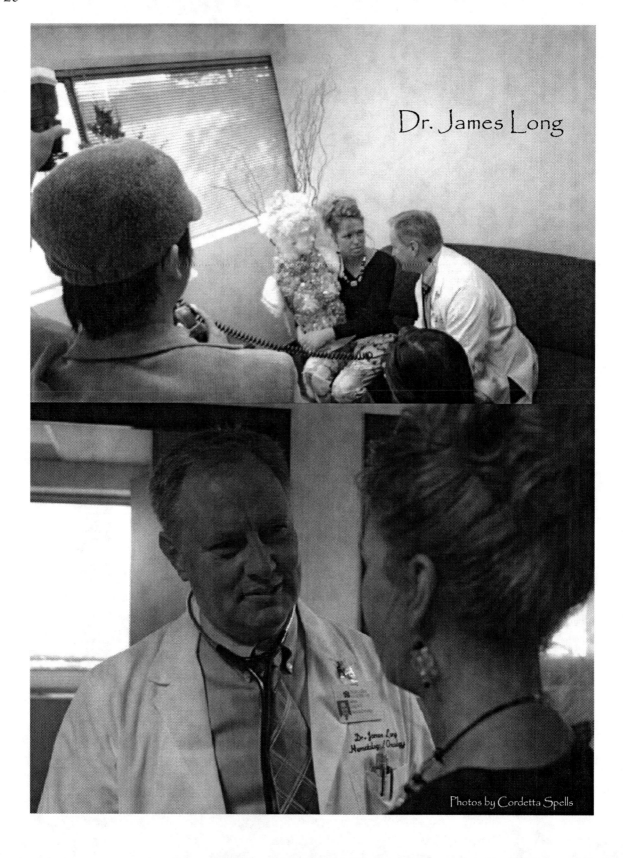

Dr. James Long

Photos by Cordetta Spells

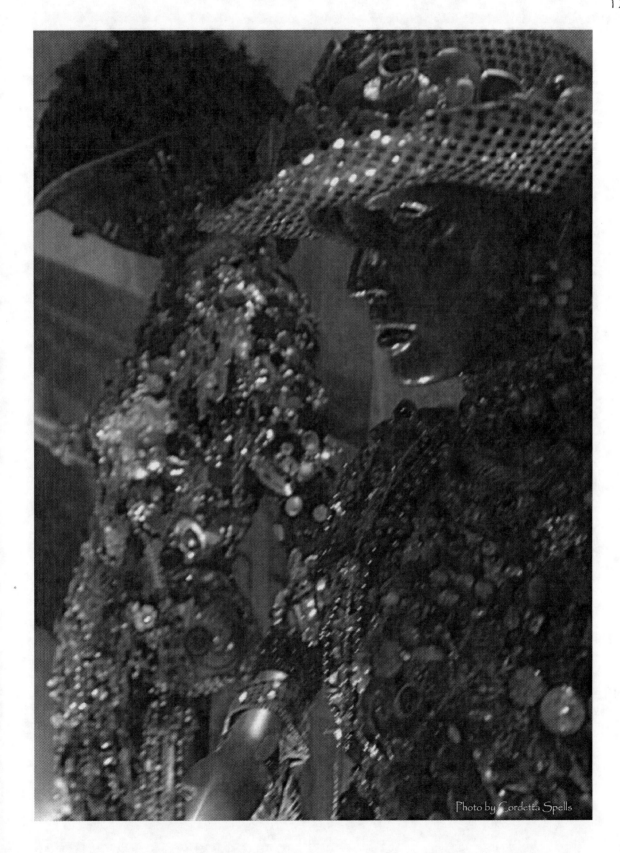

Photo by Cordetta Spells

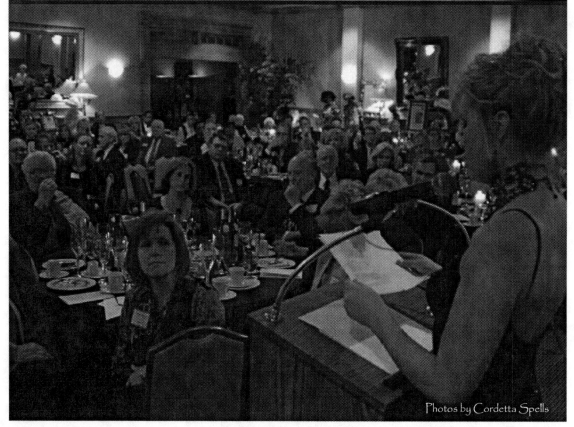

A Promising Future — Gary Passama, President / CEO, NorthBay Healthcare Corporation

Leadership Recognition and Awards Presentation — Mike Paulik, Chair, NorthBay Healthcare Foundation

Tomasini Award
Business Leadership Award
Physician Leadership Award
Employee Humanitarian Award
New Founders Circle Members
New Endowment Funds
New Legacy Circle Members

A New Legacy — Heidi Marble, Buttons-n-Dollars

Closing Thoughts — Mike Paulik, Chair, NorthBay Healthcare Foundation

Photos by Cordetta Spells

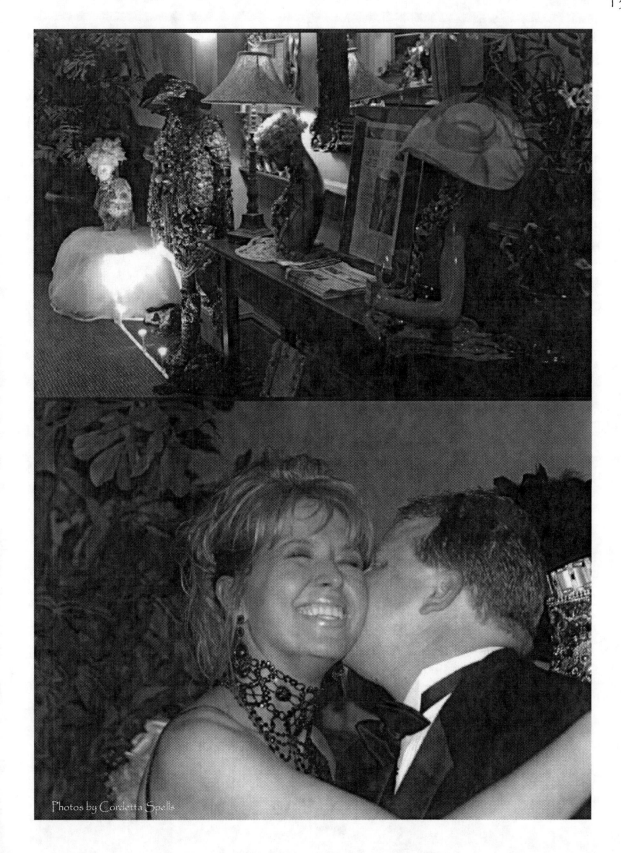

Photos by Cordetta Spells

Ezio

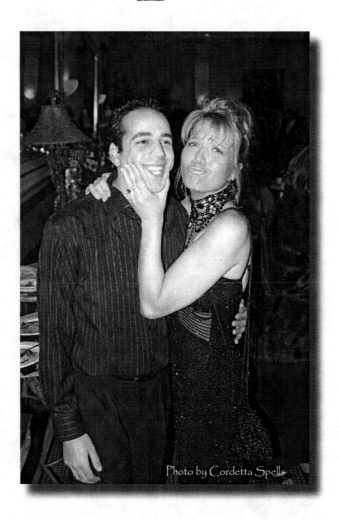

Photo by Cordetta Spells

Ezio's Documentary

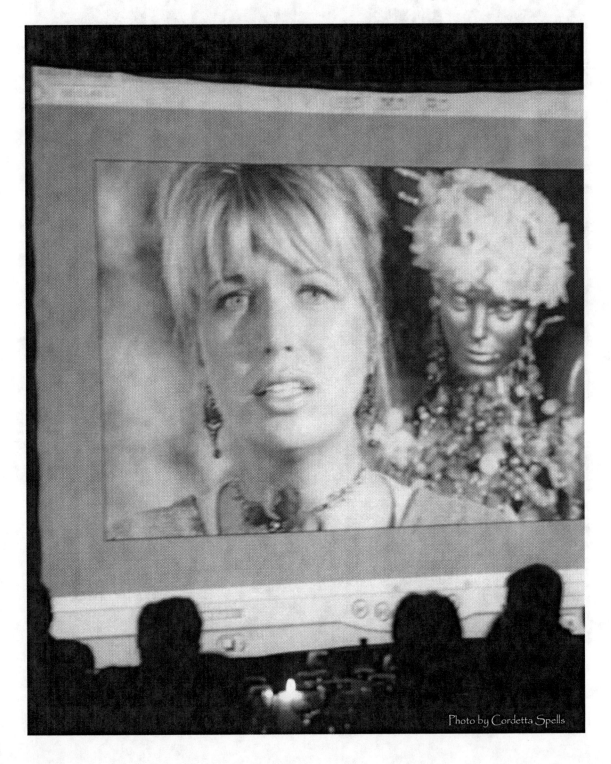

Photo by Cordetta Spells

134

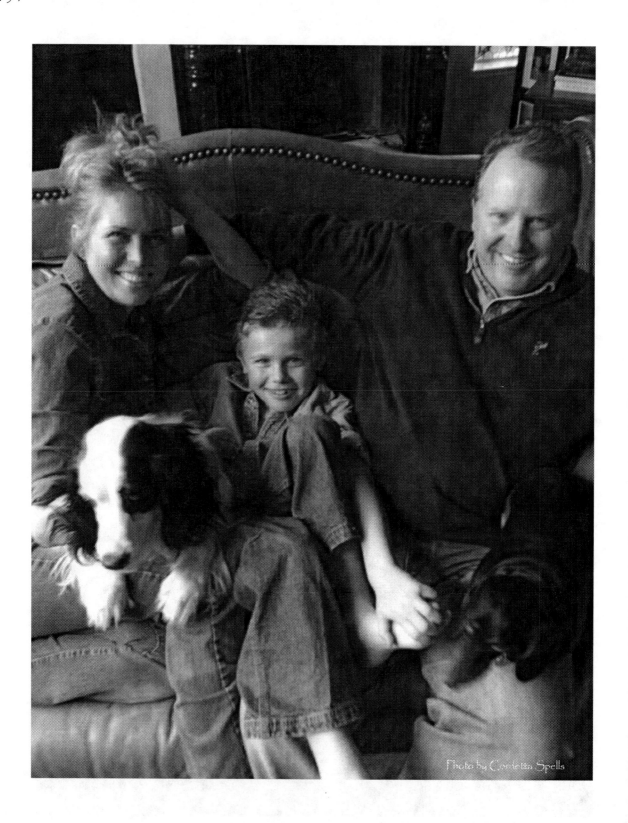

Photo by Cordetta Spells

FLUTTER, BUTTERFLY

You have found your safety among the fresh, green leaves
Your emerald chrysalis shining with dew
Emerge
Let the casing fall away
Liquefy your colors for the rainbow
Twirl with the wind that lives inside you
Glide fully open
Drink the flowers' sweetness
Let your fragility be your strength
Cherish your design and the arc of your wings
You are light and free
Flutter, butterfly
Flutter

Photo by Cordetta Spells

RESOURCE GUIDE

Here For Now
Living Well with Cancer Through Mindfulness
Elana Rosenbaum
Foreword by Jon-Kabat-Zinn
www.mindfuliving.com

After Breast Cancer
A Common-Sense Guide to Life After Treatment
Hester Hill Schnipper, LICSW
Foreword by Lowell E. Schnipper, MD

Breast Cancer Husband
How to Help Your Wife and Yourself Through Diagnosis, Treatment, and Beyond
Marc Silver
Foreword by medical oncologist Frederick P. Smith, M.D.

100 Questions and Answers About Breast Cancer
Zora Brown
LaSalle D. Leffall, Jr., MD, with Elizabeth Platt
Foreword by Senator Dianne Feinstein

The Race is One Step at a Time
Every Woman's Guide to Taking Charge of Breast Cancer & My Personal Story
Nancy G. Brinker
Founder of Susan G. Komen Breast Cancer Foundation and Race for the Cure

Coping With Cancer Magazine
www.copingmag.com

CONTACT INFORMATION

Undone (Home of Buttons-n-Dollars)
Heidi Marble
heidi@buttons-n-dollars.com
www.buttons-n-dollars.com
www.waitingforwings.com

Lifes Images Photography
Cordetta Spells
Two-time Emmy Award-winning photojournalist
lifesimages@earthlink.net

WiseWords Editing
Stephanie Parrish
language.lover@gmail.com

B&M Design Websites/Graphic Art
Eric Ball & Russ Martellaro
bandmdesign@gmail.com

Graphic Auto Body (more than your average auto body shop)
Greg Matthews
www.graphicautobody.com

Motion EclipsePictures
Ezio Lucido
Film, Video, Music, Media
elucido@motioneclipse.com
www.motioneclipse.com

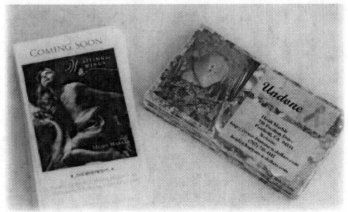

Photo by Cordetta Spells

ENDNOTE

1. Martha Diaz, "Monarch Butterfly," *Insecta Inspecta World,* 1999. http://www.insecta-inspecta.com/butterflies/monarch/index.html (accessed March 8, 2006); "Monarch Butterfly Metamorphosis Photos," *MilkweedCafe.com.* http://www.milkweedcafe.com/photos.html (accessed March 8, 2006).

Printed in the United States
93102LV00002B/1-116/A

9 781885 852465